Up

4 WEEK LOAN

This book is due for return on or before the last date shown below.

Don Gresswell Ltd., London, N21   Cat. No. 1208   DG 02242/71

Updated ENT

G.G. Browning MB, ChB, MD, FRCS(Edin), FRCS(Glas)
Professor in Otorhinolaryngology, University of Glasgow

Third Edition

A member of the Hodder Headline Group
LONDON • NEW YORK • NEW DELHI

This edition first published in Great Britain in 1994 by Butterworth Heinemann.

This impression published in 2001 by
Arnold, a member of the Hodder Headline Group,
338 Euston Road, London NW1 3BH

http://www.arnoldpublishers.com

Distributed in the USA by
Oxford University Press Inc.,
198 Madison Avenue, New York, NY10016
Oxford is a registered trademark of Oxford University Press

Whilst the advice and information in this book are believed to be true and
accurate at the date of going to press, neither the authors nor the publisher
can accept any legal responsibility or liability for any errors or omissions
that may be made. In particular (but without limiting the generality of the
preceding disclaimer) every effort has been made to check drug dosages;
however, it is still possible that errors have been missed. Furthermore,
dosage schedules are constantly being revised and new side-effects
recognized. For these reasons the reader is strongly urged to consult the
drug companies' printed instructions before administering any of the drugs
recommended in this book.

British Library Cataloguing in Publication Data
A catalogue record for this book is available from the British Library

Library of Congress Cataloging-in-Publication Data
A catalog record for this book is available from the Library of Congress

ISBN 0 7506 1921 X

1 2 3 4 5 6 7 8 9 10

Printed and bound in India by Replika Press Pvt Ltd, 100% EOU, Delhi 110 040

What do you think about this book? Or any other Arnold title?
Please send your comments to feedback.arnold@hodder.co.uk

The first edition is dedicated to Annette for being a lifelong supporter.

The second edition is dedicated to my colleagues and the otologists and scientists in particular.

The third edition is dedicated to David for just being David.

Contents

Preface to the third edition

With each edition of a successful textbook, the runs get larger. Hence the time between editions tends to lengthen and the time lapse since the last edition is now seven years. In medicine, many changes take place over such a period and this edition has been extensively revised and partly rewritten to take this into account. With time, personal interests narrow, so for this edition, I have taken advice from an even wider range of colleagues than formerly: Stuart Gatehouse, Kenneth MacKenzie, Iain R.C. Swan, Janet A. Wilson and P.J. Wormald. Hospital time is scarce so the owners and trustees of the following are thanked for allowing me to sit and rewrite this text: Grosvenor Hotel, Glasgow; Hilton Hotel, Istanbul; Meridian Hotel, Helliopolis; Cyclops Hotel, Fethiye; Paradise Hotel, Jerusalem; and Nico's.

G.G. Browning

Preface to the second edition

A text called *Updated ENT* requires to be brought up to date regularly and it is suprising what changes there have been in knowledge and clinical practice since the first edition in 1982. Thanks on this occasion are mainly due to Iain R.C. Swan, FRCS, for his helpful comments and for support as a colleague. Thanks are also due to the various owners and trustees of the following properties where, apart from my home and hospital, I have had the time to revise the book. Boston Museum of Fine Arts, Massachusetts; Cleveland Museum, Ohio; Kansas City Airport, Kansas; Queen Elizabeth Hall, London; Tate Gallery, London.

Preface to the first edition

The prime aim of medical education must be to train clinicians in the methods of arriving at a diagnosis so that the most appropriate management is applied. Many undergraduate textbooks do not take a practical approach, but simply list the various pathologies and describe their presenting signs, symptoms and management. They do not mirror bedside teaching where one is taught to elucidate a patient's symptoms and to give a number of potential diagnoses before clinical examination allows a diagnosis to be made. Students are mainly taught in Departments that slavishly investigate patients, often at great expense. This may be academically interesting, but students should be made aware that the majority of diagnoses can be made without any investigation whatsoever. Otorhinolaryngology is a specialty where it is possible to see the majority of the structures in which one is interested, although it can be difficult on occasions. Investigations are, therefore, perhaps less important than in other specialties. The main area that otolaryngologists cannot see is the inner ear and it is in this area that it is most difficult, even with investigations, to arrive at a diagnosis.

   The aim of this book is, therefore, to instruct students in how to take a patient's otolaryngological symptoms, to arrive at a diagnosis by logical steps and then to manage the problem. When one takes a 'cook book' approach it is inevitable that one will be criticized. This is valid because there are as many different ways of arriving at a diagnosis as there are of baking a cake. Students should not be surprised if what they are told in their lectures and what they are taught in the clinics is rather different from what is written here. Indeed, they would not be receiving a University education if it were to be so. It is up to them to observe and, through practice and experience, to be in a position to be able to carry out their own recipes.

My education in English is abysmal and if the text is at all readable it is because various individuals have corrected the spelling and my wife has tried to teach me to express myself clearly. Finally, I thank all my numerous colleagues for their comments on these notes and for their support in running the University of Glasgow undergraduate course in Otolaryngology, for which this text was initially written.

The ear

Anatomy and examination of the ear

The ear is divided functionally into three parts (*Figure 1.1*), the external, the middle and the inner ear, and different otological diseases affect each part.

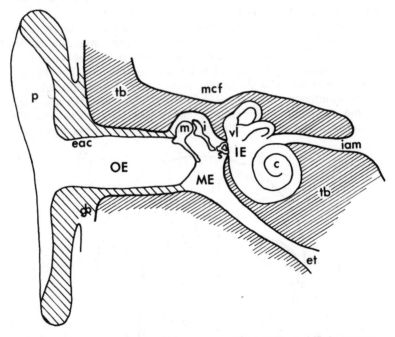

Figure 1.1 *Basic ear anatomy.* OE, outer ear; ME, middle ear; IE, inner ear; P, pinna; eac, external auditory canal; m, malleus; i, incus; s, stapes; vl, vestibular labyrinth; c, cochlea; tb, temporal bone, mcf, middle cranial fossa; iam, internal auditory meatus; et, Eustachian tube

External ear anatomy

The pinna (or external ear) and the external auditory canal are skin-covered structures and are, therefore, mainly affected by skin diseases; dermatitis (*Otitis externa*) and boils (*furuncles*) being the commonest.

However, the skin of the outer external auditory canal is different in that it also has multiple specialized sebaceous glands which secrete cerumen. This partially evaporates, and is normally shed as dry flakes along with the dead skin that naturally migrates out of the canal. *Wax retention* may occur, especially where there is a narrow canal, or where there is a surgically created mastoid cavity. Perhaps a more important factor is attempts to clear it out with proprietary cotton buds. This often does nothing but cause *wax impaction* further down the canal. The other culprit that impacts wax is the mould of a hearing aid. Though wax may prevent visualization of the tympanic membrane it does not cause a hearing impairment unless it becomes impacted deeply in the canal (page 39).

The audiological purpose of the pinna and external auditory canal is to collect sound and transmit it to the tympanic membrane. The tympanic membrane consists of a multilayered, fibrous membrane covered by a single layer of squamous epithelium. The fibrous layers are attached to the handle of the malleus, allowing sound to be transmitted to the inner ear via the ossicular chain. The main part of the tympanic membrane is called the pars tensa and the posterosuperior part is called the pars flaccida. Above this is the

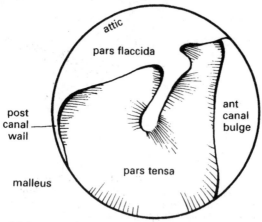

Figure 1.2 Anatomy of the right tympanic membrane

bony attic (*Figure 1.2*). Middle ear infections can affect these parts singly or in combination.

Examination of the external ear

The pinna and surrounding skin can be readily examined without instruments but preferably in good light. Operation scars can be difficult to detect because of their positioning in skin creases. Postauricular scars (*Figure 1.3*) usually indicate previous mastoid surgery and endaural scars (*Figure 1.4*) middle ear surgery, although both areas can be approached through either incision.

To examine the ear further requires illumination and a speculum to hold the external auditory canal open. Originally otologists used sunlight and silver aural speculae. The present generation use a hand-held, battery-powered auriscope with plastic speculae. An operating microscope is frequently used in specialist clinics and this

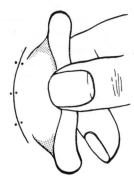

Figure 1.3 Postauricular scar

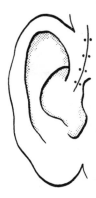

Figure 1.4 Endaural scar

allows the external auditory canal, tympanic membrane, attic and middle ear structures to be assessed accurately. However, no matter what optical system is used, as large a speculum as the external auditory canal will take ought to be used. The pinna must be pulled posterosuperiorly before the speculum is inserted so that the cartilaginous bend of the external auditory canal is straightened. This will allow the canal skin to be examined fully, as well as allowing visualization of the tympanic membrane.

Middle ear anatomy

This is an air-filled space containing the ossicular chain. The middle ear communicates anterosuperiorly to the nasopharynx via the Eustachian tube, and posterosuperiorly to the mastoid air cells via the antrum (*Figure 1.5*).

The middle ear and Eustachian tube are lined by a mucus-secreting, ciliated epithelium. The air cells are lined by a simple layer of mucosa which, when inflamed undergoes metaplasia and becomes mucus secreting. *Otitis media with effusion* is the name given to the condition when the middle ear is filled with non-infected mucus. Alternatively, the mucosa can become infected and the middle ear

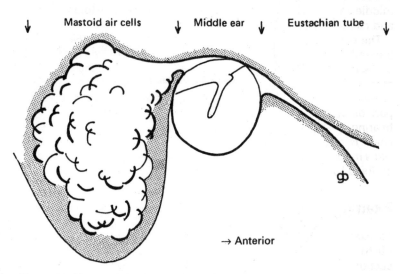

Mastoid air cells ↓   Middle ear ↓   Eustachian tube ↓

→ Anterior

Figure 1.5 Air containing connections of the right middle ear

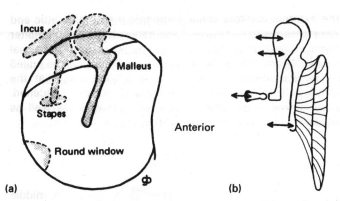

Figure 1.6 The right ossicular chain: (a) lateral view; (b) anterior view

and mastoid air cells fill with pus – *acute otitis media*. Sometimes the tympanic membrane temporarily ruptures to effect drainage. *Chronic otitis media* develops in some individuals when the tympanic membrane fails to heal because of repeated infections.

The mastoid air cells are in close relationship to the dura and the middle and posterior cranial fossae. Meningitis and intracranial abscesses can, therefore, occur by direct spread from middle ear infections. The facial nerve runs in a thin bony canal through the middle ear and mastoid before it exits via the stylomastoid foramen and can also be affected by infection.

The ossicular chain of the malleus, incus and stapes (*Figure 1.6*) transmits sound vibrations from the tympanic membrane to the fluid of the inner ear. The whole acts as a piston, the area of the tympanic membrane being considerably greater than that of the stapes footplate in the oval window. A conduction defect can occur in any part of the system. If the tympanic membrane is perforated the hearing loss is proportional to the size of the defect. If the ossicular chain is disrupted, such as at the incudostapedial joint in *chronic otitis media*, a conductive defect occurs. Alternatively the stapes can be fixed by *otosclerosis* in the oval window.

Examination of the middle ear

To examine the tympanic membrane fully requires any visually obstructing wax or pus to be removed by mopping, syringing or suction. Beginners often find it difficult to locate the tympanic membrane. This is because they tend to look in a posterior rather than anterior direction. One of the easier landmarks to the tympanic membrane is the handle of the malleus. The tympanic membrane is inspected to see if it is intact or not. If intact is it normal in appearance (*Figure 1.2*) or is it scarred and calcified; the latter indicates *tympanosclerosis* (*Figure 1.7*). It is next assessed as to whether it is in a normal position or is it retracted due to *negative middle ear pressure* or *otitis media with effusion* (*Figure 1.8*). Alternatively it may be bulging and inflamed due to middle ear pus

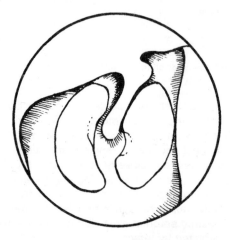

Figure 1.7 Tympanosclerosis of right tympanic membrane

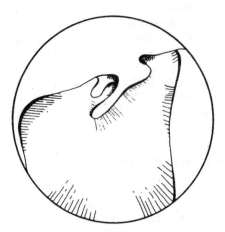

Figure 1.8 Otitis media with effusion (right ear)

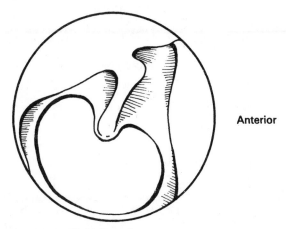

Anterior

Figure 1.9 Chronic otitis media (right ear)

under tension in *acute otitis media*. If the tympanic membrane is not intact it will usually be because of a perforation associated with *chronic otitis media* (*Figure 1.9*). The site of the perforation can be anterior, posterior, inferior or a combination. The proportion of the tympanic membrane that is defective can also be assessed. If there is a perforation it should be possible to see the middle ear mucosa through it. If it is pale and dry the diagnosis is *inactive chronic otitis media*. If it is inflamed, oedematous and producing mucus or pus the diagnosis is *active chronic otitis media*. See Flow Chart 1.

The attic area above the tympanic membrane should always be examined, particularly where there is an aural discharge, in order not to miss attic disease, especially a cholesteatoma.

An open mastoid cavity in the posterosuperior canal wall is too often missed. Such a cavity results from the surgical treatment of chronic otitis media where mastoid infection needs eradicating and the risk of intracranial infection needs reducing. Hence the presence of a postauricular scar should alert the examiner to the possibility of a cavity. How a cavity is created is best understood by comparing a diagram of the normal ear (*Figure 1.10*) with a diagram of a modified radical mastoidectomy (*Figure 1.11*). The disease is drilled out of the mastoid air cells and the resultant cavity is opened into the external auditory canal by removing the posterior canal wall.

Every clinician should be able to examine the external auditory canal and tympanic membrane but it is usually left to otolaryngologists to examine the Eustachian tube orifices in the postnasal space

OTOSCOPY

Examine the pars tensa and pas flaccida separately after removing wax, debris and pus. Examine open mastoid cavity if present.

PARS TENSA

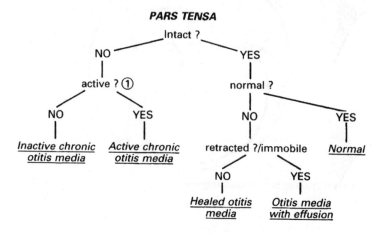

PARS FLACCIDA

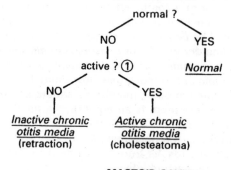

MASTOID CAVITY

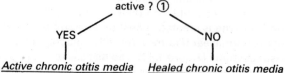

Note ① Activity indicated by presence of mucus/mucopus in external auditory canal with inflamed oedematous middle ear mucosa

Flow Chart 1 Otoscopy

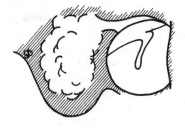

Anterior

Figure 1.10 Normal anatomy (right ear)

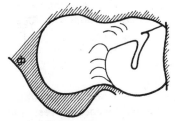

Anterior

Figure 1.11 Modified radical mastoidectomy created by removing the posterior canal wall

with the aid of a mirror or a nasendoscope. On the other hand, there is no reason why every clinician should not be able to determine if the Eustachian tubes are functioning by assessing the mobility of the tympanic membrane. This can be done by altering the middle ear pressure, either by the patient performing a Valsalva manoeuvre or, if they cannot do this, by the clinical use of a pneumatic auriscope.

The object of a *Valsalva manoeuvre* is to increase the pressure in the postnasal space, whence, if the Eustachian tube opens, it is transmitted to the middle ear, causing the tympanic membrane to move. The patient is therefore instructed to:

1. Take a deep breath.
2. Close off their nose by pinching it shut.
3. Shut their mouth.
4. Exhale, keeping their nose and mouth shut.
5. If their ears are normal, the patient should then feel them 'pop'.

Children, and many adults, often find the above instructions difficult. They can usually be persuaded to blow up a balloon with their nostril with the same effect (page 48).

The clinician is, of course, looking at the tympanic membrane during this manoeuvre. If the tympanic membrane moves there is no need to do anything further. Failure of the tympanic membrane to move is most frequently due to the failure of the patient to relax their soft palate and, therefore, the Eustachian orifices are shut off. Get them to do it again and this time to swallow whilst trying to exhale against a closed mouth and nose.

If the procedure is performed correctly there are two pathologies that can be associated with an immobile tympanic membrane. The first is a small perforation that has been missed. The second is middle ear fluid associated with *otitis media with effusion*. Because of the unreliability of patient performance, it is wise to try and move an immobile tympanic membrane actively with a pneumatic oto-scope. With such a system, the external auditory canal is hermet-ically closed off with the speculum, and the pressure in the canal is varied by pressing a small air bulb which is connected to the system.

Inner ear anatomy

Functionally, this is divided into the cochlea and the vestibular labyrinth (*Figure 1.12*), which are supplied by the cochleo-vestibular (VIII) nerve.

Cochlea

After arriving at the oval window, sound vibrations are transmitted in the perilymph compartments of the cochlea to the hair cells on the

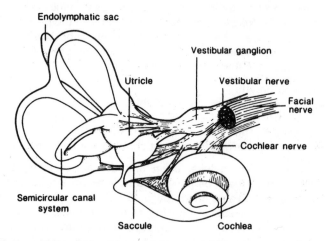

Figure 1.12 The vestibular system. This shows the relationship within the temporal bone of the endolymph containing vestibular system, its innervation by the vestibular nerve and the cochlea

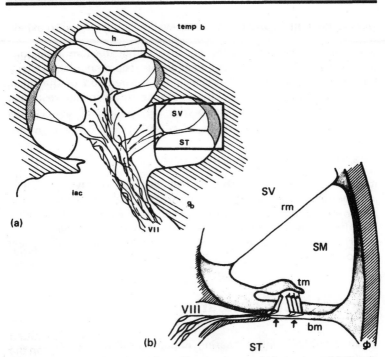

(a)

(b)

Figure 1.13 (a) *Section through cochlea to show spiral structure.* (b) *Blow up of boxed area to show details.* bm, basilar membrane; tm, tectorial membrane; rm, Reissner's membrane; SM, scala media; ST, scala tympani; SV, scala vestibuli; h, helicotrema; iac, internal auditory canal; temp b, temporal bone; VIII, cochlear nerve; ↑, point to hair cells

basilar membrane which winds up the bony spiral of the cochlea (*Figure 1.13a*). This allows sound frequency discrimination to occur because of differential vibration along its length. The high frequencies stimulate the base of the cochlea, and this is the region most commonly damaged in a sensorineural hearing impairment. From the hair cells, nerve impulses pass along the cochlear division of the VIII (auditory) cranial nerve (*Figure 1.13b*) which runs in the internal auditory canal along with its vestibular division and with the VII (facial) cranial nerve. It then joins the brain stem, interconnects with nerve fibres from the other side, and passes up to the higher cerebral centres. It is in the internal auditory canal that the VII nerve can be affected by an *acoustic neuroma* (page 54) or a *temporal bone fracture* (page 175).

Vestibular labyrinth

The sense organs of balance are also within the temporal bone (*Figure 1.12*). The three semicircular canals record angular acceleration and the saccule and utricle linear acceleration of the head. Neurological impulses from these organs travel in the vestibular division of the VIII nerve, along with the cochlear division, to the brain stem.

Examination of the inner ear

It is not possible to do this directly because of the inner ear's inaccessibility. Radiology, and in particular computerized tomography, define the anatomy well and can be used to decide whether it is affected by disease. However, in most patients, the diagnosis of inner ear disease is by the exclusion of external or middle ear pathology.

Clinical tests of hearing

In an individual with a hearing impairment four aspects require evaluation.

1. **Severity of the impairment** This is done clinically by free field speech testing, and audiometrically by pure tone audiometry.
2. **Type of impairment** The impairment can be conductive, sensorineural or mixed, i.e. both. The distinction is primarily made by otoscopically detecting a conductive pathology or by pure tone audiometry. Tuning fork tests may sometimes be of help.
3. **Pathology causing the impairment** Clinical examination of the ears will usually identify conductive pathologies, but tympanometry can be useful in the diagnosis of otitis media with effusion. The aetiological factors responsible for a sensorineural hearing impairment are usually suspected from the history.
4. **Disability caused by the impairment** This is assessed by questioning the patient and by observing the patient in the clinic.

Free-field speech testing

To establish the threshold of hearing the patient is asked to repeat, as accurately as possible, words that are spoken to him. The point at which the patient repeats approximately half of the words correctly is the threshold.

Since there are two ears to be evaluated, it is necessary to mask the hearing in the non-test ear. One method of doing this is to occlude the external auditory canal by placing a finger on the tragus and then rubbing the tragus in a rotary manner. Alternatively, a clockwork noise box (Barany box) can be used but this is usually unnecessary unless there is a gross inequality in the hearing between ears, or if the hearing impairment is marked.

In order to assess the threshold of hearing there are two ways of varying the loudness of the voice. The first is the distance from the test ear: 6 inches is as close as one might wish to go, and 2 feet is as far away as one can stretch whilst masking the non-test ear. Secondly, the level of the voice can be varied from a whisper to a normal conversational level and then to a loud voice.

The words which the patient is asked to repeat should not be easy to guess; numbers like 99 or 44 are too easy. Either bisyllable words such as cowboy or hatrack or a combination of numbers and letters such as 9B5 or C3U are preferable.

After explaining to the patient to repeat as best he can the words that are said to him, the clinician stands behind rather than in front of him to obviate speech reading, masks one ear and starts off with a simple word so that the patient understands what is required. A normal individual in a quiet room should easily hear test words in a whispered voice at arm's length (2 feet). Indeed a normal hearing individual should easily hear a whisper at 18 feet but this is difficult to assess unless someone masks the other ear for the examiner. It is important to use a whisper and not just a quiet voice. In a whisper the vocal cords do not vibrate and the words are just mouthed. This is most easily achieved by exhaling before whispering. If the patient cannot hear a whispered voice at arm's length, then he has a hearing impairment. Further testing by increasing the relative sound inten-

Table 1.1 Thresholds of hearing

Voice level	Distance	Impairment
Whisper	2 feet	Normal
	6 inches	Mild
Conversation	2 feet	Moderate
	6 inches	Moderate
Loud	2 feet	Severe

sity of the voice until the patient can repeat what is being said will assess the magnitude of the impairment. The threshold of hearing is that distance and voice level at which the ear can hear at least 50 per cent of the test words (*Table 1.1*). The other ear is then tested in a similar manner.

Rinne tuning fork test

This tuning fork test may help to determine whether hearing impairment has a conductive component to it. It does not help to determine whether there is a hearing impairment, this is achieved by free-field speech testing.

The basis of this test is that the normal ear hears sounds louder via the external auditory canal and middle ear (air conduction) rather than directly through the skull (bone conduction). However, if a defect occurs in any part of the conduction mechanism of the external canal or middle ear then the air conduction can appear quieter in comparison with the bone conduction. Thus, if the tympanic membrane is perforated or the ossicular chain disrupted then the bone conduction may appear louder than the air conduction (Rinne negative).

If the impairment is purely sensorineural then air conduction will still appear louder than bone conduction (Rinne positive). It is unfortunate that in many instances when there is a material conduction defect the air conduction will still be louder than the bone conduction. As such it is emphasized that the most reliable way to determine whether there is a conductive defect or not is to compare the bone conduction thresholds with the air conduction thresholds on pure tone audiometry (page 16).

Method

A tuning fork with a frequency of 256 or 512 Hz is normally used. This is activated either by pressing the prongs together or by lightly hitting them on the elbow.

The activated tuning fork is first held close to the external auditory meatus with the prongs in line with the canal and the patient is asked if he can hear the sound. The base of the fork is then pressed on the skull posterosuperior to the ear and the patient is asked if he can hear the sound and whether it is louder or quieter than when the fork was held at the external auditory meatus. If a patient cannot decide which is louder, the level of the sound from the fork, held at the external auditory meatus, is allowed to decay until the patient can no longer hear it. If the patient then hears the sound when the fork is placed on the skull, bone conduction is better than air conduction.

Interpretation

If the bone conduction is louder than the air conduction (Rinne negative) there is likely to be a conduction defect. If the air conduction is louder than the bone conduction, there may be no impairment (i.e. normal) or the impairment may be sensorineural, conductive or mixed (*Figure 1.12*).

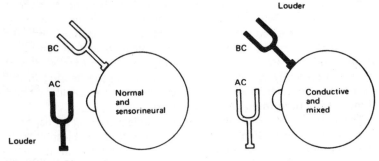

Figure 1.14 Rinne test

■ Conclusions

- The presence or a hearing impairment is determined by free-field speech testing.
- If an individual cannot hear whispered words at arm's length then he has a hearing impairment.
- The severity of a hearing impairment can be graded by free-field speech testing at the distance and voice level at which words are repeated correctly.
- The Rinne tuning fork test may determine whether there is a conductive component to a hearing impairment. This is suggested if the bone conduction sounds louder than the air conduction.
- The most reliable way to determine whether an impairment is sensorineural, conductive or mixed is by pure tone audiometry, provided this is reliably performed with appropriate masking.

Audiometry

Audiometry can do several things more accurately than clinical tests of hearing. It can assess whether there is a hearing impairment and, if there is one, its severity and what proportion of it is due to a conduction defect as opposed to a sensorineural defect. On occasions it can also help to identify the aetiology of an impairment. Whether the results can be relied upon depends on several factors. Some relate to how and where the assessment was carried out and to whether the patient was cooperative.

It might seem obvious that to assess the hearing accurately the test has to take place in a sound-deadened room or booth so that extraneous noise will not affect the hearing but it is surprising how often tests are carried out in less than ideal circumstances. Another variable is the tester's ability to carry out the tests and, in particular, to use masking. Because sound readily goes round the skull and even more readily vibrates through it, masking the hearing in the non-test ear is essential. Suffice it to say that this can be difficult and if incorrectly performed will lead to errors.

The majority of tests rely upon the subject making a response such as whether he heard the sound or not. Such subjective tests depend upon the patient being able to comprehend what he has to do and then doing this to the best of his ability. When this is not the case, such as in infants or individuals exaggerating their hearing impairment to claim compensation, objective tests are required. The reason that objective tests are not used all the time is that they are time consuming and use expensive equipment.

Subjective tests

Pure tone audiometry

The patient is told to respond whenever he hears a sound. By lowering and raising the sound level at which pure tones of different frequencies are presented the thresholds of hearing can be assessed both by air and bone conduction. It is generally held that when the average air conduction thresholds are 25 dB HL (Hearing Loss) or poorer over the four speech frequencies (0.5, 1, 2 and 4 kHz) there is an impairment (*Figure 1.15*). If the air and bone conduction thresholds are similar the impairment is sensorineural (*Figure 1.16*). If the bone conduction thresholds are better than the air conduction thresholds, as evident by an air–bone gap of greater than 10 dB, there is a conductive defect (*Figure 1.17*).

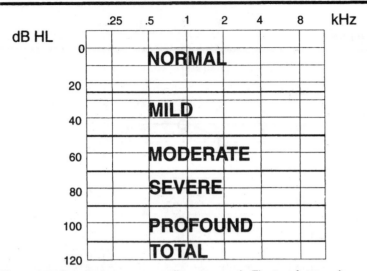

Figure 1.15 Standard pure tone audiometry graph. The test frequencies are at the top on the horizontal axis and the degree of impairment in dB HL (Hearing Loss) is on the vertical axis. The further down the chart a patient's threshold lies, the poorer the hearing. This particular graph is divided into bands of different degrees of hearing impairment, e.g. a patient with an average threshold between 50 and 70 dB HL has a moderate impairment.

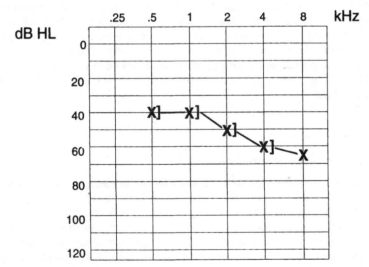

Figure 1.16 Left-sided sensorineural impairment (left air conduction x, left bone conduction])

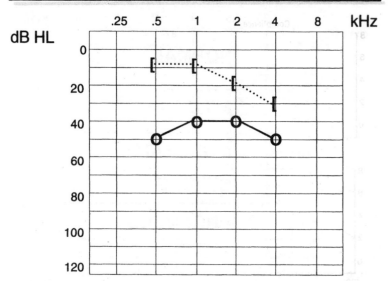

Figure 1.17 Right-sided conductive impairment (right air conduction o, right bone conduction [)

Speech audiometry

The subject is asked to repeat back the words which are presented to him at various sound levels. This assesses the severity of the impairment and perhaps even more importantly assesses the subject's disability in understanding speech. There are many individuals with a sensorineural impairment who can never score 100 per cent of the words correct no matter how loud the volume is turned up.

Objective tests

Electric response audiometry

If repeated sound signals are presented to the ear, it is possible with electrodes and by computer averaging techniques to pick up the electrical responses to these in the cochlea (electrocochleography), in the brain stem (brain stem evoked responses) or in the cerebral cortex (slow vertex) and separate them out from other neurological, electrical activity. The thresholds of hearing can be assessed and, by analysing how quickly the responses arrive, it can be suggested where in the auditory pathway the pathology might be.

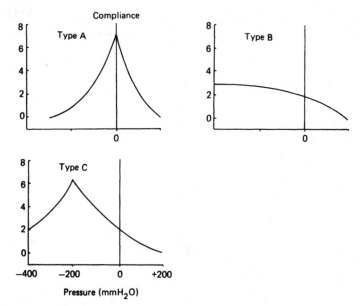

Figure 1.18 *Classic tympanograms.* Type A, normal; Type B, middle ear fluid; Type C, negative middle ear pressure

Impedance audiometry (tympanometry)

The test ear is sealed off with a probe which has three ports in it: one to change the pressure in the external auditory canal, another to introduce sound and another to a microphone which measures how much sound is absorbed. Most sound is absorbed when the external auditory canal pressure is the same as that in the middle ear. So by varying the pressure, graphs of compliance are obtained whose peak indicates the middle ear pressure. A normal graph has its peak around $0\,mmH_2O$. Negative middle ear pressure is indicated by a shift of the peak to the negative side. Fluid in the middle ear is indicated by an absent peak (*Figure 1.18*).

■ Conclusions

• Accurately performed audiometry is more reliable than clinical methods in assessing the severity of an impairment and deciding whether it is conductive or sensorineural.

- Audiometry is not without its technical difficulties, the most important of which is the masking of the non-test ear.
- Pure tone audiometry is the standard method of assessing hearing thresholds.
- In those who cannot or will not respond accurately, electric response audiometry is an objective but less accurate alternative.
- The decision as to whether an impairment is conductive or sensorineural rests on a comparison of the air and bone conduction thresholds on a pure tone audiogram.
- Impedance audiometry may help diagnose negative middle ear pressure and otitis media with effusion.
- Electric response audiometry can help to determine where in the auditory pathway any pathology is present.

The commoner inflammatory pathologies

The nomenclature used to describe the commoner inflammatory conditions that affect the external auditory canal and middle ear is numerous, overlapping and confusing to the uninitiated. The conditions also present in different ways, so in this symptom-based text each will be included under several different headings. The following is an overview of each condition, with its synonyms, pathology, aetiology and symptomatology in order of frequency of the mode of presentation.

Otitis externa

Synonyms

Dermatitis/eczema of the external auditory canal.

Pathology

Non-specific inflammation of the skin and subcutaneous tissues of the canal causing oedema and increased epithelial desquamation.

Aetiology

Essentially unknown and likely to be a combination of the following:

- Decreased skin defence barrier.
- Trauma, e.g. from cotton bud, finger, match, etc.

- Climate/environment. Hot sweaty damp conditions.
- Allergy to poking instruments, e.g. nickel in pins.
- Bacteria colonizing an already inflamed epithelium.
- Iatrogenic. Secondary irritation to chemicals and eardrops. Secondary allergy to topical antibiotics. Fungal infection secondary to topical antibiotics.

Presenting symptomatology

- Ear discomfort/itch.
- Ear discharge.
- Mild hearing impairment.

Acute otitis media

Synonyms

Suppurative; purulent; bacterial otitis media.

Pathology

A bacterial infection of the middle ear and mastoid air system which occurs primarily in infants and young children. Spontaneous resolution usually occurs sometimes with rupture and drainage through the tympanic membrane. Very rarely the drainage of pus from the mastoid air cells becomes blocked with the development of an abscess within the mastoid – mastoiditis. In addition, because of its proximity the infection can spread to the dura causing meningitis or brain abscess.

Aetiology

- Viral upper respiratory infections.
- Poor Eustachian tube function due to a combination of the age of the child and oedema secondary to the upper respiratory infection.
- Bacterial infection – usually with mixed, upper respiratory tract flora. Mainly streptococci, staphylococci, pneumococci and *Haemophilus influenzae*.
- Genetic/environment: commoner in the lower socio-economic groups.

Presenting symptomatology

- Otalgia.
- Pyrexia/malaise.
- Sometimes aural discharge.

- Very rarely with the complications of meningitis, brain abscess or mastoiditis.

Otitis media with effusion

Synonyms

Serous otitis media, secretory otitis media, glue ear.

Pathology

Non-specific inflammation of the middle ear mucosa associated with non-draining of the resultant mucus down the Eustachian tube.

Aetiology

Unknown but likely to be a combination of the following:

- Recurrent upper respiratory tract infection.
- Repeated episodes of acute otitis media.
- Close contact with other children, especially at school.
- Poor Eustachian tube function.
- Adenoid hypertrophy.
- Parental smoking.

Presenting symptomatology

- Hearing impairment.
- Otalgia.

Chronic otitis media

Synonyms

Chronic suppurative otitis media.

Pathology

The primary pathology is chronic inflammation of the middle ear and mastoid air cell mucosa which results in permanent loss of at least part of the tympanic membrane giving a chronic perforation. There may be erosion of part of the ossicular chain, most commonly at the incudostapedial joint. Secondary hyalinization and sometimes ossification (tympanosclerosis) can occur in the remaining fibrous layers of the tympanic membrane and the suspensory ligaments of the ossicles giving an added conduction defect. The mastoid air cells become progressively obliterated by fibrosis and new bone growth.

The course of chronic otitis media is variable. In some the activity is intermittent with the production of muco-pus. In some it becomes burned out and inactive. Sometimes the vestibular labyrinth is involved giving vertigo. On a rare occasion, the disease causes a facial nerve palsy or spreads intracranially to cause meningitis or a brain abscess.

A variant of active disease is where there is in association a cholesteatoma which is a squamous epithelial lined retraction pocket with a narrow neck which causes it to retain epithelial debris.

Aetiology

Unknown but thought to be a combination of:

- Previous acute otitis media.
- Previous otitis media with effusion.
- Poor Eustachian tube function.
- Recurrent upper respiratory infection including sinusitis and bronchitis.
- Bacterial infection.
- Genetic/environment: commoner in the lower socio-economic groups.

Presenting symptomatology

- Hearing impairment.
- Frequently an aural discharge.
- Sometimes vertigo.
- Rarely with the complications of facial palsy, meningitis or brain abscess.

Otosclerosis

Synonym

Otospongiosis.

Pathology

New bone growth mainly in the oval window area. Females are more likely to get secondary stapes fixation than men.

Aetiology

Genetic predisposition otherwise unknown.

Presenting symptomatology

• Hearing impairment, unilateral or bilateral of a conductive type.
• Normal, mobile tympanic membrane.

Runny ears

As in many conditions, the history and clinical examination can be diagnostic for a patient with an aural discharge (*See Flow Chart 2*). The main differential diagnosis is *wax, otitis externa* or *active chronic otitis media*. Acute otitis media is not included as its presenting symptom is otalgia rather than an aural discharge which only occurs in some. The following two questions are usually helpful in deciding the most likely pathology.

What is the discharge like?

A discharging ear means different things to different patients so the clinician must elicit its real nature. Some patients consider soft wax to be a discharge but obviously this is not so. However, contrary to industrial folklore, a smelly discharge is abnormal and is a sign of inflammation in the external auditory canal or in the middle ear. On occasions a mucopurulent discharge may be mixed with blood and this is most often due to the inflamed mucosa in active chronic otitis media being traumatized by a cotton bud.

Otitis externa and otitis media can usually be distinguished by the following question.

Is there an associated itch or discomfort?

If an itch or aural discomfort is present this is usually diagnostic of otitis externa. The itch makes the patient want to scratch or poke the ear and this type of discomfort can usually be distinguished from otalgia (page 32). In chronic otitis media there is rarely otalgia because the chronic tympanic membrane perforation does not allow the middle ear pressure to build up.

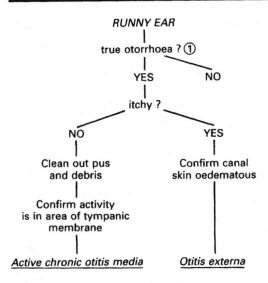

RUNNY EAR
|
true otorrhoea ? ①
|
YES   NO
|
itchy ?
NO   YES
| |
Clean out pus   Confirm canal
and debris   skin oedematous
|
Confirm activity
is in area of tympanic
membrane
|
Active chronic otitis media   *Otitis externa*

Note ① Ensure discharge is not wax and is watery/smelly and perhaps stains pillow.

Flow Chart 2 Runny ear

These initial questions are usually all that are necessary to arrive at a diagnosis which can then be confirmed otoscopically. Further questions can be asked later after assessing the ear.

How to examine the ear

Look for operation scars

Postauricular and endaural scars (*Figures 1.3, 1.4* page 3) should be visible if looked for closely.

Look at the external ear

Otitis externa often affects the auricular skin as well as that of the external auditory canal.

Press the tragus

In severe otitis externa pressure will cause discomfort, whereas in chronic otitis media it will not.

Look in the external auditory canal

At this stage it is most likely that the discharge will be seen. Syringing (page 69) is probably the most efficient way to clean out the entire canal so that the tympanic membrane can be seen. In this instance there is no need for concern regarding syringing an ear with a perforation as the ear is already infected. The alternative is to assiduously mop out the canal with cotton buds. Once the ear has been cleaned the following should be done.

Look at the canal skin

In otitis externa the skin will be red and glazed and the canal will often be narrowed by oedema and fibrosis.

Look postsuperiorly

To see if there is a mastoid cavity (*Figure 1.11*, page 9) and, if this is present, whether it is clean or full of debris and infected material. If full of debris, clean it out either by mopping, syringing or with suction, if available.

Look at the tympanic membrane

The handle of the malleus, and especially its lateral process, is usually the easiest structure to recognize and from which to

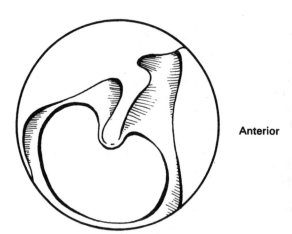

Anterior

Figure 1.19 Right tympanic membrane perforation

establish landmarks. The tympanic membrane is then inspected to see whether it is intact. If in doubt, use a pneumatic auriscope (page 47). If the tympanic membrane is intact it will be seen to move. In active chronic otitis media a rounded perforation of the pars tensa (*Figure 1.19*) can usually be detected once the pus has been mopped away. Through the perforation it is often possible to see inflamed middle ear mucosa. Sometimes granulation tissue or, more rarely, a polyp arising from the middle ear obscures the view.

In active chronic otitis media an alternative site of the disease is the attic. The inflammation here is usually associated with a retraction pocket of squamous epithelium which becomes filled with debris (*Figure 1.20*). This is what is called a *cholesteatoma*.

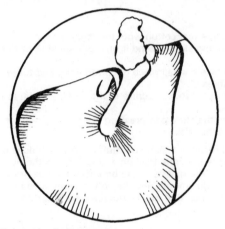

Figure 1.20 Right attic cholesteatoma

In conclusion, if the ear is properly cleaned out it is usually possible, taking into account the history, to distinguish between otitis externa and active chronic otitis media as the cause of a discharging ear. It is wise at this stage to test the hearing clinically by using free-field voice testing (page 12).

Having made the diagnosis what do you do next?

As far as the basic management is concerned, it does not matter what the diagnosis is; aural toilet is essential in both otitis externa and active chronic otitis media. For the non-specialist syringing is

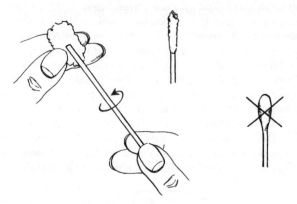

1. Get some real cotton wool (not synthetic) and
   something slim to wind it on – orange stick or florist
   wire.
2. Then take a small piece of cotton wool and tease out
   the fibres.
3. Place tip of stick in centre of the wool, parallel to the
   fibres.
4. Rotate the stick, compressing the fibres around the
   top of the stick.

The end result is a slim soft, fluffy bud which does not
come off with gentle traction and which has the tip of
the stick in the middle of the bud. (Sometimes orange
sticks are too smooth and the cotton wool does not grip
well. A rougher end can be obtained by breaking the
stick).

Figure 1.21 Instructions for making a cotton bud

preferable to mopping with cotton buds. Commerial buds are large,
hard and tightly wound. They can be teased out to be slimmer and
fluffier so that they are easier to insert and are more absorbent. The
alternative is to make them oneself (*Figure 1.21*) but many find this
difficult. However, specialists use these regularly, making them on a
Jobson Horne probe. They then mop out under direct vision via a
speculum using a microscope or head light. Non-specialists usually
cannot do this and may damage the ear. The majority of patients
with otitis externa and many with chronic otitis media will respond
symptomatically to aural toilet alone. Many clinicians prefer a 'belt
and braces' approach so additional treatments can be given, most
frequently topical medications.

Specific management of otitis externa

Aural toilet, plus if required:

1. *Topical ear preparation* to soothe and medicate. A large variety of preparations are available including steroid (hydrocortisone, betamethasone, or dexamethasone), glycerol and ichthamol or aluminium acetate. Antibiotics should not be included in steroid preparations for otitis externa as any organisms present are commensals or secondary invaders rather than the cause of the disease. Topical antibiotics often make the otitis externa worse by causing an allergic skin reaction or superinfection with bacteria and fungi. How topical preparations are used depends on several factors.
    a. *Drops* are slightly difficult for the patient to use (see below) but a wide variety of medications are available in this form.
    b. *Ointments and creams* can be applied on the canal skin by fine cotton buds or squeezed from the tube directly into the ear.
    c. *Sprays* are easy for the patient to use and, provided the canal is not too narrow and has been cleaned of debris, have a very good surface distribution. Unfortunately only steroid and antibiotic sprays are currently available.
    d. *Wicks* are used if the external auditory canal is too narrow. Impregnate a ½-inch ribbon gauze wick with an ointment or cream and insert as far as possible into the canal. This will allow the canal to open up and topical preparations on their own can then be substituted. In some this will fail and insertion of wicks by a specialist may be required.
2. *Analgesics* if discomfort is not controlled with topical applications.
3. *Exclude irritants and allergens.* It is natural to poke an itchy ear but sometimes the tool is sharp and traumatizes the canal skin. Cotton buds are the only thing to use. Ear drops to soften wax can irritate and thus be a cause of otitis externa.

Failure to respond to treatment is usually due to inadequate removal of debris from deep in the meatus.

Non-specialist management of active chronic otitis media

The majority of patients will require specialist assessment at some stage because chronic otitis media, as long as it is active, is an unsafe disease. This is because complications are common. The hearing can deteriorate because of ossicular chain erosion or cochlear damage.

Vertigo can develop because of irritative labyrinthitis or semicircular canal fistulae. Mastoiditis, facial palsy, meningitis and intracranial abscess can also occur but fortunately less frequently.

Thus although the non-specialist can initiate management, this will only be of short-term benefit, if at all, in eliminating the activity. In the majority, activity is episodic or continuous and the long-term management is surgery. It is only the rare patient who develops activity in a normally inactive ear, for example following swimming. Even in them there will be a hearing impairment due to the tympanic membrane defect which may benefit from surgical repair.

Non-specialist management pending referral

1. *Aural toilet.* The patient should be instructed in how to clean out their external auditory canal with cotton buds, either teased out commercial buds or self-made if the patient can do so. They should be encouraged to put these in as far as possible having pulled the pinna posterosuperiorly to straighten the canal. No damage will be done unless it is painful. Mopping should be repeated until the cotton buds come out dry and this should be done at least three times per day. Children and some adults find mopping difficult so parents or nurses may have to do this for them. Moping will lessen the ear discharge and hence the patient will symptomatically improve. However, in most cases the ear will remain active and topical medications are required in addition.

2. *Topical steroids and antibiotic eardrops.* These cannot be given without first mopping the ear as the medication has to make contact with the inflamed middle ear mucosa and this will not occur unless the pus has been removed. A variety of preparations are available which include chloramphenicol, clioquinol, framycetin, gentamicin and neomycin along with steroids. Some would suggest caution with the use of aminoglycosides in these preparations because of the theoretical risk of ototoxicity. Topical antibiotics on their own are valueless as are systemic antibiotics. Instilling preparations requires the head to be held in a lateral position for 2 or 3 minutes so that the drops reach the middle ear. Positive displacement is achieved by intermittently pressing the tragus whilst in that position. Because of the ease of use and better topical distribution, spray medications are likely to displace drops in the future.

3. *Specialist referral.* This is urgent if the patient has any serious complications such as vertigo. It is important also in those that have recurrent episodes of discharge and those with a significant hearing impairment.

Specialist management of active chronic otitis media

Otolaryngologists will usually perform:

1. *Microsuction and mopping* under direct vision usually with a microscope to fully clean out the ear and assess the extent and type of the disease. In particular, they will differentiate between active mucosal disease and cholesteatoma.
2. *Audiometry* will accurately record the magnitude of any conduction defect and the severity of the impairment in both ears.
3. *Surgery* following discussion with the patient as to the objectives; to dry the ear, prevent complications and perhaps improve the hearing. For active mucosal disease the crucial factor is to graft the tympanic membrane (myringoplasty). Any ossicular chain abnormality may be repaired then or at a second stage operation (tympanoplasty). For cholesteatoma it is usually necessary to drill to expose the disease (atticotomy) and, if this is found to be extensive, to open the mastoid into the posterior canal wall and create an open mastoid cavity (modified radical mastoidectomy).

■ Conclusions

- Otitis externa and active chronic otitis media are the main causes of a discharging ear.
- The history of the type of discharge and the presence or absence of itch or pain are usually diagnostic.
- The ear will require thorough aural toilet before being examined.
- Clinical examination is also diagnostic.
- Whichever the cause, aural toilet by mopping, syringing or both is essential.
- In otitis externa this may be all that is required. Topical preparations, e.g. steroids applied by sprays or drops if the canal is open or by wicks if closed may be of additional benefit.
- In active chronic otitis media the majority of sufferers should have a specialist otolaryngological opinion.
- Non-specialist management is topical steroids and antibiotic sprays or drops in addition to mopping.
- Specialist management usually includes surgery.

Pain in the ear

It can be difficult to elucidate the cause of a painful ear, mainly because the pain can originate locally in the ear or temporomandibular joint, or it can be referred from elsewhere in the head and neck. This is because the trigeminal (V) and glossopharyngeal (IX) nerves have a considerably greater area of innervation than the ear *Figures 5.8* and *5.9* page 166). Otological conditions are generally associated with other otological symptoms, most frequently by examining the ear. Temporomandibular causes can almost always be identified by eliciting tenderness over the joint and on straining the jaw. If no otological or temporomandibular pathology is identified then it must be referred pain.

The diagnostic possibilities for otalgia are different in children and in adults. Therefore they will be dealt with separately.

Otalgia in children

Perhaps the commonest type of history is of a young child, usually under the age of 3, waking in the middle of the night screaming and crying with earache. Often there is a history of a preceding cold or cough and the differential diagnosis is acute otitis media, otitis media with effusion, negative middle ear pressure or referred pain from the teeth, or the upper respiratory and alimentary tracts. To make a distinction is not easy and rests mainly on otoscopy. As the mainstay of management irrespective of the cause is analgesics such as paracetamol elixir, a degree of uncertainty as to the diagnosis is not too relevant within the first 24 hours. In the majority the pain will have resolved by that time but if it persists then an accurate diagnosis becomes important (see Flow Chart 3).

Acute otitis media

Here the otalgia is due to a build-up of pus under pressure within the middle ear. The diagnosis is made by finding a bulging, red inflamed tympanic membrane. Lesser degrees of redness are common in the crying child without acute otitis media and can cause diagnostic difficulties. In these cases the drum will not bulge and will be mobile on pneumatic otoscopy.

The primary management is analgesics with the addition of antibiotics (ampicillin, amoxycillin), particularly if the child is systemically unwell as evident by fever and/or lymphadenopathy.

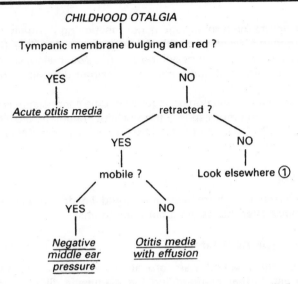

Note ① An otologic cause for the child's otalgia is unlikely.
Consider pharynx and teeth.

Flow Chart 3 Childhood otalgia

Antibiotic therapy is by no means mandatory, no major benefit having been demonstrated in controlled trials. In most children, the pain settles rapidly within several hours due to spontaneous resolution or less frequently by rupture and drainage of pus via the tympanic membrane. Some would suggest that antibiotics be reserved for children in whom the condition persists and certainly such children required to be followed up in an effort to abort potential complications such as meningitis and mastoiditis. If these are suspected, hospital management is mandatory.

All children who have had acute otitis media should be reviewed about 6 weeks later to assess their hearing as some will proceed to have otitis media with effusion.

Negative middle ear pressure/early otitis media with effusion

Though the majority of children with chronic middle ear effusion do not have otalgia, it can sometimes occur. The reasons for this are as follows. Otalgia is only caused by sudden changes in the differential pressure across the tympanic membrane between the middle ear and the external auditory canal. So in the diagnostic situation being described the Eustachian tube is not functioning normally because of the oedema associated with the upper respiratory infection. The child is sleeping, mouth breathing and not swallowing, so the air is absorbed from the middle ear and a painful differential pressure develops.

The otoscopic detection of negative middle ear pressure is difficult at any time, and more so in a fretful child. Pneumatic otoscopy can be helpful. Crying should not be discouraged as it can help to get air back into the middle ear.

Teething

The referred pain from teething should be detected by eliciting tenderness over the, as yet, unerupted tooth.

Upper respiratory infection

Pain from the inflamed naso-, oro- and hypopharynx can be referred to the ear, further confounding the diagnostic dilemma. It is by excluding otological and teething problems that the diagnosis is made.

Otalgia in adults

Though the conditions that cause otalgia in children can also cause it in adults they are relatively infrequent compared with the following.

Otitis externa

The diagnosis should be evident by otoscopy and the management is as described elsewhere (page 29).

Boils

These can be acutely painful and sometimes difficult to distinguish from severe otitis externa. Local heat and analgesics are usually all that are necessary.

Negative middle ear pressure

The aetiology of this, as in children, can be an upper respiratory infection but frequently there is the added insult of changes in atmospheric pressure associated with air travel or diving.

Temporomandibular joint inflammation

This is almost always associated with major gaps in the dentition, loose dentures or non-wearing of dentures, which all cause continued strain on the joint. The joint itself will be tender to palpation and pain will be caused by opening the jaw and shoving it to one side. The long-term management is by providing better dentition. In the short term, anti-inflammatory analgesics are useful.

Cervical osteo-arthritis

Pain due to this can usually be elicited by rotating and/or laterally positioning the head. X-rays are of minimum value as many older spines will be osteo-arthritic anyway. Management is with anti-inflammatory analgesics and perhaps neck rest with a cervical collar.

Pharyngeal tumours

Though uncommon in comparison with the other causes of otalgia in adults, it is a diagnosis not to be missed. There may or may not be other symptoms expected to be associated with such tumours (page 121). Unfortunately, the presence of pain with such tumours usually indicates involvement of the glossopharyngeal nerve at the base of the skull and therefore a poor prognosis, however treated.

■ Conclusions

- Otalgia is as frequently non-otological (due to referred pain) as it is otological in origin.
- Otological conditions are usually diagnosed by otoscopy. If none are present it is most likely referred pain and a cause for this should be looked for.
- In children the commoner otological causes are acute otitis media, negative middle ear pressure and otitis media with effusion.
- In children the commoner non-otological causes are discomfort from the naso- and oropharynx associated with an upper respiratory tract infection or with teething.
- In adults, otitis externa, boils and negative middle ear pressure following air travel or diving are the main otological causes.
- In adults, temporomandibular and cervical joint problems are the common non-otological causes. A naso- or oropharyngeal neoplasm is a rarer possibility.

Hearing impairment in adults

In the region of 20 per cent of adults have a hearing impairment, the higher proportion being sensorineural. The high prevalence of sensorineural impairments is mainly related to age, not that age itself is the cause, it is rather that the chances of being exposed to the factors that cause impairments increase with age. It is surprising how many older patients do not complain spontaneously of having hearing difficulties. This is probably due to a combination of the slowly progressive nature of most impairments and the expectation that the hearing will naturally deteriorate with age. The clinician should, therefore, train himself to anticipate and identify hearing problems rather than waiting for patients to complain. Though patients often attribute their impairment to wax this is usually not the case. Impacted wax can on occasions cause an impairment but it is usually an additive, rather than the only, cause.

As sudden hearing losses present differently and are considered an otological emergency, they are considered elsewhere (page 54).

How to arrive at a diagnosis

A patient who complains of difficulty in hearing probably has! The elucidation of its cause requires a combination of a clinical history and examination. The history will identify any aetiological factors which might be responsible for a sensorineural impairment. Free-field voice testing will confirm the presence of an impairment. Otoscopy will identify the majority of conditions that cause a conductive impairment, the main exception being otosclerosis where the tympanic membrane will be normal. The history will also indicate the situations where the patient is disabled, which is important for management, as this is tailored to each patient. Pure tone audiometry is usually performed to confirm the severity and type of the impairment but the patient's disability is by no means directly related to the pure tone audiogram.

History

The order in which the following questions are asked will depend on how a patient responds, but answers to them all should be known at the end of the examination.

How much trouble is the patient having in hearing?

The disability that a patient has in hearing not only dictates the need for management but in many instances its form. It is necessary to ask the patient this question because disability is not directly related to the severity of the impairment as measured by voice testing or by an audiogram. This is for many reasons but not least the ability of the patient to overcome a disability by speech (lip) reading. Often the earliest evidence of an impairment is listening to conversation in a noisy background. With more severe impairments there will be difficulty in hearing in a 'one to one' conversation, listening to the television and using the telephone. Whether the patient has a particularly bad side should be noted as this indicates asymmetric hearing. It is not uncommon for a patient to attribute all his hearing difficulties to one ear when in reality they have a bilateral impairment with one poorer ear. As sound readily travels round the skull it is the degree of impairment in the better hearing ear that mainly determines the degree of disability. The exception is in a noisy situation and a speaker is on the side of the poorer speaking ear.

What is the natural history of the impairment?

Most impairments usually affect both ears and slowly progress over many years, but occasionally the impairment comes on suddenly. Hopefully, if this occurs, a patient will be referred to an otolaryngologist as soon as possible for investigation and management (page 54). Another type of impairment is one that fluctuates and, in the absence of other symptoms or obvious factors such as water, this is almost certainly due to otitis media with effusion.

Is one ear worse than the other?

The commonest reason why an individual might have a unilateral or asymmetric impairment is that there is a conductive defect in the poorer ear. To disregard this is not of great concern, but to disregard a unilateral or asymmetric sensorineural impairment can be dangerous because one of the causes of this is an acoustic neuroma.

Are there any associated symptoms?

It should be ascertained whether a patient has tinnitus, vertigo, otalgia or an aural discharge and, if present, further enquiries are as indicated elsewhere.

Are there any obvious aetiological factors?

Do the ears run?
The presence of a smelly discharge, without pain or discomfort, suggests active chronic otitis media, but it is surprising how many patients with an ear full of pus state that the ear does not run.

Have they been exposed to noise?
Everyone today is exposed to unnecessary noise but this is usually of little consequence. The levels that should cause concern are those at work which make communication difficult, as exemplified by the need to shout. The risk of damage is related to the number of years of exposure but the risk can be virtually eliminated by the wearing of ear muffs or plugs. In any patient with an impairment their job history should be enquired about and a note also made about impact noise such as rivetting, machine stamping and shooting, as these produce a sensorineural impairment more readily than constant noise. Although disco music is loud enough to have an effect on hearing, most people are not exposed for a sufficient total number of hours for this to have a permanent effect.

How is their general health?
Many generalized diseases are thought to have an effect on hearing. The cochlea is supplied by an end artery and is likely to be subject to the effects of both peripheral and general vascular disease. Thus, a history of diabetes, strokes, transient ischaemic attacks, angina, myocardial infarction, hypertension and intermittent claudication would all support an ischaemic factor in the impairment.

What drugs are they on?
This follows on naturally from the previous question. Many drugs have been suggested to cause or aggravate an impairment, in particular, aspirin, beta-blockers, loop diuretics and cisplatinum. Unfortunately, the only drug-induced impairment that is totally reversed by stopping the drug is aspirin.

The aminoglycosides are considerably more likely than anything else to cause an impairment but the mode of onset is sudden, is often associated with vertigo, and is usually clearly related to its prescription.

Clinical examination

By the time the history has been taken it will usually be fairly obvious whether communication with the patient is difficult or not. Inability to communicate should not be automatically ascribed to senility or idiocy. Although this is sometimes the case, it is surprising how much more alert a patient can become once he or she has been fitted with a hearing aid.

There is no set routine to the clinical examination but the experienced clinician will also have noted automatically, while taking the history, whether the patient is speech (lip) reading. The next thing to do is to test the hearing, especially if there is uncertainty as to whether the patient has an impairment or not. This is done by free-field speech testing (page 12). Having confirmed that there is indeed an impairment the next thing to do is examine the ears. Flow Chart 4 is a suggested flow pattern used to arrive at a diagnosis.

Are there any operation scars?

This alerts the clinician to the likelihood of the pathology being chronic otitis media and prevents him from automatically ascribing anatomical abnormalities to a disease process.

Is there obstructing wax?

Wax is secreted in the outer third of the canal and though it will frequently obstruct the view of the tympanic membrane it is infrequently the cause of an impairment. This is because sound traverses the external auditory canal as vibrations, so provided the wax can vibrate in the column of air it will not cause an impairment. It is only when the wax is impacted into the deeper canal against the tympanic membrane, most frequently by attempts to clean it out with cotton buds or by the repeated insertion of the mould of a hearing aid that it is likely to cause an impairment (*Figure 1.22*).

If the tympanic membrane cannot be seen the wax ought to be removed (page 69) because the majority of conductive pathologies are diagnosed by otoscopy. Once the wax has been removed the hearing should be retested, and it is only if the impairment has been eliminated that wax can be said to have been its cause.

DIAGNOSIS OF HEARING IMPAIRMENT

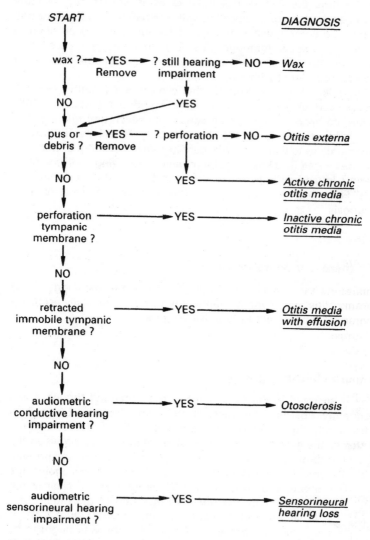

Flow Chart 4 Simplified flow diagram of the means of arriving at a diagnosis of the cause of hearing loss by clinical examination

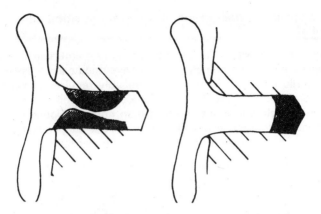

Figure 1.22 The wax in the ear in the left diagram would not cause a hearing impairment whereas the wax on the right would do so

Is there any pus, mucus or debris?

If there is any, it has to be removed (page 69) so that a full evaluation can be made. Pus and/or debris in the external auditory canal implies one of two diagnoses. In cases where the skin of the canal is thickened, tender to the examining speculum and produces some degree of canal narrowing, the diagnosis is otitis externa. If there is a tympanic membrane perforation with a mucopurulent discharge the diagnosis is active chronic otitis media.

A patient may have otitis externa secondary to the pus from active chronic otitis media, so it is vital to visualize the whole area of the tympanic membrane and the attic. To do this requires thorough aural toilet to remove all the pus either by mopping or syringing.

Is the tympanic membrane intact?

Chronic otitis media can, of course, be inactive and there will be no pus or mucus in the canal or middle ear, but there will be a perforation of the tympanic membrane or a defect in the attic. The tympanic membrane may be intact but have white plaques of calcification within it, leading to a diagnosis of tympanosclerosis, which is the end result of any form of otitis media. If the tympanic membrane is intact there remain two relatively common causes of a conductive impairment, otitis media with effusion and otosclerosis. The two are distinguished by the answer to the next question.

Is the tympanic membrane in a normal position and mobile?

In otitis media with effusion the tympanic membrane is usually retracted due to a combination of negative middle ear pressure and the middle ear fluid. To detect this reliably requires considerable experience but is best detected by looking at the handle of the malleus which will be less vertical than normal (*Figure 1.23*). The tympanic membrane itself will look more cone-shaped and perhaps bluish or yellow in colour due to the middle ear fluid.

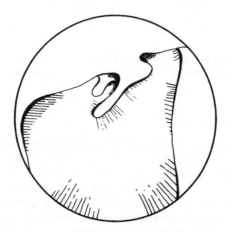

Figure 1.23 Otitis media with effusion. Note the retracted, preshortened handle of the malleus compared with normal (*Figure 1.2*)

Another way to diagnose otitis media with effusion is to assess whether the tympanic membrane is mobile. This can be evaluated either dynamically or passively. Watch the tympanic membrane while the patient performs a Valsalva manoeuvre (page 9). If the tympanic membrane moves, the Eustachian tube is patent and there is no fluid in the middle ear. If the tympanic membrane does not move it could be that the patient cannot perform a Valsalva manoeuvre. Positive pressure can then be applied to the external auditory canal by pressing the bulb of a pneumatic auroscope while observing the tympanic membrane. If the tympanic membrane does not move then the diagnosis is otitis media with effusion. Tympanometry (page 19) essentially does the same thing mechanically and can in many cases be helpful in confirming the diagnosis.

What type of hearing impairment is it?

Although the commoner causes of a conductive impairment should have been identified at this stage by otoscopy, tuning fork tests (page 14) can be performed which may help determine whether the impairment has a conductive component to it. However the only way reliably to determine the type and severity of the impairment is by pure tone audiometry. In the presence of a normal external auditory canal and tympanic membrane, a conductive impairment is most likely to be due to otosclerosis, with congenital abnormalities or ossicular disruption being the alternatives. To distinguish between these is sometimes not easy.

If the impairment is of a sensorineural type, there is little apart from the history to distinguish between the various aetiological factors (*Table 1.2*). An important exception is an acoustic neuroma where further audiometric and radiological tests are of value (page 53).

Table 1.2 Aetiological factors responsible for sensorineural impairments

Bilateral impairments	Unilateral impairments
Idiopathic (age)	Idiopathic
Noise trauma	Trauma (including surgery) Viral infections (mumps and measles)
Genetic	Meningitis Vestibular syndromes (including Ménière's) Acoustic neuroma

How to manage a hearing impairment

Each patient is managed as an individual, and how this is done will depend on the patient's age, general health, lifestyle, degree of disability in varying situations, the type of hearing impairment, its presumed aetiology and the presence of other symptoms. In general, almost all hearing impairments can be helped by a hearing aid (page 60) and if there is a conductive component, surgery may also be of benefit. The next section deals with the specific management of the few sensorineural conditions that can be managed and with the surgical management of the commoner conductive pathologies. The management of other symptoms is dealt with elsewhere.

Specific management of hearing in sensorineural impairments

Noise trauma

Impairments due to noise exposure are irreversible, so management is to prevent further exposure. The easiest way to do this is to avoid excessive noise altogether but this is often impractical especially for those at work or in the armed forces.

The issue of ear 'defenders' is now compulsory in certain industries where there is a high level of noise but employees often pay no heed and go unprotected. There is little evidence that wearing defenders makes communication with other workers difficult and this argument for non-wearing should be refuted. There are many other situations where ear defenders should be worn. For example, all pneumatic drills and power chain saws have a high noise output and some older tractors and lorry drivers' cabs are extremely noisy. The crucial factors in the creation of a hearing loss are the noise level, whether there is sudden impact noise, and the length of time exposed.

The methods of protection are head muffs or ear plugs (either of insulating cotton, foam or malleable plastic). Ear plugs offer less protection than muffs, and cotton wool is useless.

Ototoxic drugs

As soon as a drug is implicated as being a possible aetiological factor it should be stopped. This applies particularly to the aminoglycosides (gentamicin, kanamycin, streptomycin, etc.) and cisplatinum where some recovery of hearing can take place. There should be no difficulty in substituting an alternative drug from a different generic group.

Acoustic neuroma

Surgery, via the ear or the middle or posterior cranial fossa, is necessary to prevent an acoustic neuroma growing and causing intracranial compression. Surgical complications are considerably less for small tumours, so early diagnosis is in the patient's interest. Unfortunately, the hearing usually has to be sacrificed but as the other ear is often normal this is not too disabling. A facial palsy can also occur as it is often difficult to avoid damaging it during surgery.

Specific management of conductive hearing impairments

Chronic otitis media

The tympanic membrane defect can be repaired using fascia from the adjacent temporal muscle. In appropriate hands, such myringoplasties are highly successful in both improving the hearing and preventing further activity. If the ossicular chain is defective it can be rebuilt using either the patient's own ossicle or an autograft of cartilage or bone. Artificial prostheses are less satisfactory. Again in the correct hands, such tympanoplasties (i.e. myringoplasty with ossiculoplasty) can be very beneficial. There is no reason why these operations cannot be carried out in ears that are active but in them the surgical eradication of the inflammation usually takes precedence.

Otosclerosis

Microsurgery does not remove the otosclerosic focus but overcomes the stapes fixation by removing it in whole or in part and replacing it with a stainless steel or Teflon piston.

In the correct hands, the results are highly satisfactory. The potential complications are a sensorineural impairment, either partial or total, and disequilibrium.

There is no reason why the impairment cannot be managed with a hearing aid.

Otitis media with effusion

Many adults have dullness of hearing for a short period of time following an upper respiratory tract infection. This requires no treatment apart from auto-inflation (Valsalva manoeuvre). In a few patients the condition is chronic, lasting more than 3 weeks, and the majority of these are idiopathic in origin, perhaps being associated with chronic rhinitis, sinusitis or bronchitis. In a few it is the presenting symptom of a nasopharyngeal tumour, so referral to an otolaryngologist to exclude this is mandatory in those with chronic effusions.

Management is initially medical by any combination of auto-inflation frequently aided by a nasal balloon (page 48), systemic or topical decongestants and antibiotics. Subsequent surgical management is myringotomy with or without the insertion of a ventilating tube (grommet).

■ Conclusions

- Not all individuals with a hearing impairment are aware that they have one.
- The history is useful in identifying factors which may be responsible for a sensorineural impairment.
- Sensorineural impairments are the commonest type and the commonest identifiable factor is noise exposure.
- Otoscopy should identify the common causes of a conductive impairment, the exception being otosclerosis where the tympanic membrane is normal.
- Although wax often blocks the view of the tympanic membrane, it is an uncommon cause of a hearing impairment.
- The management of a hearing impairment is specific for each patient and depends on its aetiology and the associated disability.
- In general, sensorineural impairments are managed by amplification.
- Conductive hearing impairments can be managed by micro-surgery, amplification, or both.

Hearing impairment in children (otitis media with effusion)

At least a third of children between the ages of 1 and 8 years have recurrent episodes of otitis media with effusion more commonly called glue ear (page 22). The peak incidence is between 2 and 4 years and the main symptom is a hearing impairment. Indeed, in this age group otitis media with effusion is the only diagnosis to consider if a congenital or acquired sensorineural impairment can be ruled out (page 50). The detection of a hearing impairment can be difficult and many children with the condition go undetected. In the majority this is not serious because it resolves spontaneously without any long-term sequelae. However it is considered important to identify the few in whom it persists. This is done by paying attention to concerned parents, following up all children that have had acute otitis media and in the UK by sweep testing of all children on entry to primary school. Coincidentally, the latter is also designed to identify the rare child with a congenital sensorineural impairment which, because of its unilateral or mild to moderate severity, has previously escaped detection.

Relevant history

Parental and often grandparental concern should be listened to. They will often report that it is not so easy to attract the child's attention, and when talked to they are not so attentive. Obviously if a child has other otological symptoms such as otalgia, attention will be drawn to their ears.

The aetiology of the effusion is multifactorial but a major determinant is repeated upper respiratory tract infections. These tend to be commoner in boys and in those in close contact with sibs or other children, especially at playgroup, nursery or primary school. In about 10 per cent of children with acute otitis media the fluid fails to resolve and progresses to a chronic effusion. It is thus important to follow up such children 8 to 10 weeks after the acute episode and perform otoscopy and assess their hearing.

Non-specialist assessment and management

Otoscopy and, if the child's age makes it practicable, informal free-field speech testing of hearing are the mainstay of assessment. The appearance of the tympanic membrane is variable and coming to a firm diagnosis can be difficult. Retraction due to the negative surface tension of the effusion is usual and frequently made more obvious by an alteration in the angle of the handle of the malleus (*Figure 1.23*). Sometimes the effusion will cause a change in the colour of the tympanic membrane making it more yellow or blue. Immobility on altering the canal pressure with a pneumatic auriscope can help make the diagnosis, but tympanometry is superior and when available to the non-specialist, the finding of a flat tympanogram confirms the diagnosis (page 19).

Free-field speech testing of the hearing can be problematical but if the child is willing to talk to the examiner and can answer questions whispered from behind them, this excludes those with a bilateral hearing impairment (page 12).

Children in whom an effusion is suspected require to be followed up so that those that do not resolve spontaneously can be referred for specialist assessment. The suggested follow-up period is 6 weeks during which time medical therapy can be given. Unfortunately, nasal and systemic decongestants, antihistamines, mucolytics and antibiotics which are the commoner drugs given, have not been shown by randomized controlled trials to hasten resolution. Auto-inflation, by nasally blowing up a balloon via a plastic nose

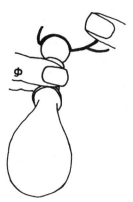

Figure 1.24 Auto-inflation with a nasal balloon

piece (*Figure 1.24*) is becoming an increasingly popular alternative to give during this observation period.

When reviewed, if the fluid persists or if there is doubt about the hearing, onward referral is recommended.

Specialist assessment and management

Though otolaryngologists will have differing degrees of concern about the various symptoms and signs of otitis media with effusion, the dominant one is the likelihood that a prolonged, bilateral hearing impairment could lead to a delay in speech and language development, as well as education. To what degree and for how long a child has to be impaired for this to occur is not yet known, but most would suggest that a bilateral impairment of 25 dB HL or poorer for 3 months could be material. Hence most would monitor the hearing over such a period. The audiometry techniques to do this should be available in all centres to test children of all ages. Testing can be time-consuming hence the initial assessment by otoscopy and/or tympanometry as to the continued presence of fluid can ease the test load by excluding those children in whom the effusion has resolved.

During the specialist monitoring period, management similar to that available to the non-specialist can be instituted. If, on reassessment, bilateral fluid associated with a documented hearing impairment persists most would then proceed to surgery.

The insertion under a general anaesthetic of a ventilation tube (grommet) after aspiration of the effusion through a myringotomy incision will improve the hearing (*Figure 1.25a* and *b*). These tubes act

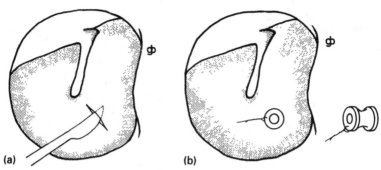

Figure 1.25 (a) Myringotomy (right ear). (b) Grommet inserted in myringotomy slit

by taking over from the Eustachian tube until the condition resolves rather than by allowing the effusion to drain through them. Adenoidectomy can have an additive effect and is often performed at the same time. Unfortunately ventilation tubes can lead to secondary infection in a third of ears and in about 5 per cent this can lead to a small permanent perforation. Swimming does not influence the incidence of infection though some continue to advise against this sport as long as the ventilation tubes are *in situ*. The time a tube will stay functioning in the tympanic membrane varies but most will be extruded spontaneously between 6 and 12 months later. This matches very closely the average time for natural resolution of the condition, but if this is not the case a tube is usually reinserted.

■ Conclusions

- In effect, the only diagnosis for a hearing impairment which develops in a previously normal hearing child is otitis media with effusion.
- The peak incidence is in preschool children and in some is a sequela of acute otitis media.
- A considerable number of children with hearing impairment go undetected and routine school screening is designed to detect these.
- The otoscopic diagnosis of otitis media with effusion can be difficult but rests upon the finding of a dull, retracted, immobile tympanic membrane.

- Tympanometry is more objective than otoscopy and where available can be used to monitor the condition.
- The most important thing is to assess clinically the hearing by free-field voice testing.
- In the majority, otitis media with effusion resolves spontaneously with no sequelae.
- Medical therapy would not appear to hasten this natural resolution.
- Auto-inflation is cheap, does no harm and gives the impression of activity.
- In those that fail to resolve and have a hearing impairment which potentially might impair their development, myringotomy and aspiration with the insertion of a ventilating grommet is the surgical management.
- Adenoidectomy may be performed at the same time.
- Grommets are associated with an increased rate of middle ear infection which is not affected by whether the child goes swimming or not.
- Grommets extrude spontaneously after about 6 months by which time the otitis media will have resolved in most children. Sometimes the grommet leaves a scar or tympanic membrane perforation.

Hearing impairment in infants

Unfortunately, hearing impairments in infants often go unrecognized, and because of the resultant sensory deprivation they can develop speech, educational and psychological problems. The main aim of those involved must be to identify infants with an impairment as early as possible so that their residual hearing can be aided by amplification and hopefully with this the child will develop normal speech and be able to lead a relatively normal life.

An infant may be either born with a hearing impairment or may acquire it early in life. When the impairment is present at birth it can be prenatal, perinatal or postnatal in origin. Such impairments will not be obvious at birth, so it is necessary to look for them. Overall the risk is about 1 per 1000 births so for practical reasons more, but not exclusive, attention is paid to infants particularly at risk, for example, because of a family history, craniofacial abnormalities or having a reason to be in a neonatal intensive care unit following birth.

Prenatal factors

The vast majority of infants with a genetically determined hearing impairment have no obvious congenital defect. They are thus not so easy to detect as the smaller group in which the impairment is part of a syndrome complex with multiple, often visible, defects (e.g. Klippel–Feil, Turner's). Children of deaf parents are obviously more at risk but in the majority, the impairment can only be attributed to spontaneous mutations.

It is normally assumed that a hearing impairment present at birth is genetic in origin if there are no other obvious factors.

The most important non-genetic, prenatal aetiology are virus infections, most commonly rubella (German measles), of the mother during the first 12 weeks of pregnancy. This is the time during which the fetal ear (otocyst) is developing and is, therefore, particularly at risk. At present, rubella cannot be treated, but it is currently recommended that all 14-year-old girls should be immunized unless they already have high antibody titres.

Cytomegaloviruses have also been suggested as a possible cause passed on from the mother. Unfortunately, unless viral titres are carried out at birth it is impossible to prove this as a cause. Drugs taken during pregnancy can cause fetal abnormalities including a hearing impairment and should, therefore, be avoided whenever possible.

Perinatal factors

In general it is a combination of factors during birth that is responsible. In particular the premature, underweight infant is particularly at risk from hypoxia, jaundice and infections. Hence screening of those admitted to a neonatal intensive care unit will identify at least a third of all infants with a severe bilateral impairment. Those given aminoglycosides whilst they are there are at even greater risk.

Postnatal factors

Postnatal sensorineural impairments are most often caused by one of three infections: mumps, measles or meningitis. Of these meningitis is associated with a higher incidence of severe impairments so all children with bacterial meningitis should have their hearing tested once they have recovered. Some consider that subclinical infection by mumps or measles viruses may also be responsible for a number of cases when no other factor can be identified.

How do you identify an infant with a hearing impairment?

Neonatal screening

The ideal would be to screen all newborn infants before they leave hospital but to do so requires some objective test, as informal observations such as the 'startle reflex' to sound are unreliable. Oto-acoustic emissions or brain stem responses to sound are reliable but relatively expensive. The alternative and relatively effective method is only to screen those at risk because of a family history, craniofacial abnormalities or having been in an intensive care unit. This will be cheaper but still identifies 50 per cent of impaired infants. Sadly in many hospitals no screening is carried out at all.

Postnatal screening

In the UK it is routine for all children to be sent an appointment for developmental checks, which include the hearing. These are usually carried out by health visitors in child health clinics. In most instances the mother will recognize that there is something wrong in the first few months of life, when the child does not respond to her voice. In addition, at this age children should be beginning to say monosyllables such as 'ba' and 'da'. It is only when children are 6–7 months old that they can be screened by using distraction tests. These are random noises, preferably generated from a portable sound box, which are presented out of sight whilst the child's attention is being held. The hearing child should turn in response to the sounds. As can be imagined, this is liable to misinterpretation and whenever there is any doubt the child should be referred to a paediatric audiology department. Here distraction testing will be repeated under stricter conditions and any impairment detected will usually be confirmed by more objective audiometry.

Children who are not babbling loudly by the age of 9 months or responding to familiar words such as their name by 12 months should be considered to have a hearing impairment. By the age of 18–30 months a normally hearing child should be able to perform cooperation tests such as responding to 'where are your shoes?' Only when the child is about 30 months old is it possible to do performance tests such as play audiometry, in which the child is taught to perform a task such as putting a brick on a pile when they hear a sound. As can be imagined, there are many children, especially those with multiple defects, in whom there is no clear answer. For them, objective tests of hearing, including evoked response audiometry, are increasingly being used.

Having identified an impairment, what do you do?

Even though the impairment may have a conductive component due to a congenital abnormality of the external or middle ear, the initial management in all cases is amplification with a hearing aid and specialized education as soon as the impairment is detected. Special high power aids are usually necessary. Acceptance of the wearing of these is better in infants than in school-age children. Regular specialist follow up is essential not only for psychological support but to ensure that the aid is being worn and not faulty. The earmoulds have to be regularly replaced because as the child grows they become ill-fitting and cannot be used at a high enough gain because of feedback.

The main aim is to integrate deaf children into the community, so if it is not possible to integrate the child totally into a normal class, the trend is to have a special class for the deaf in a normal school rather than to have separate schools for the deaf.

■ Conclusions

- It is vital to diagnose hearing impairments in infants early so that the resultant speech, communication, educational and psychological handicap can be mitigated by amplification and intensive education.
- It is better to oversuspect and thereby not miss an infant with an impairment rather than to underdiagnose.
- Audiometric testing is difficult in infants, and increasing reliance is being placed on objective methods such as evoked oto-acoustic emissions or brain stem audiometry.

Unilateral sensorineural hearing impairment

The presence of a hearing impairment in only one ear, or the presence of a hearing impairment more severe in one ear than the other, is relatively common in individuals with a conductive hearing impairment. The reason for such asymmetry usually presents no diagnostic problem.

What is less common is a unilateral or an asymmetric sensorineural hearing impairment. It is important to identify these because one of the causes, albeit a rare one, is an acoustic neuroma of the VIII cranial nerve in the internal auditory canal. Although these are benign fibromas of the nerve sheath, if left untreated they can expand outside the canal and cause death by pressure on the brain stem. It is, therefore, important to identify an acoustic neuroma as early as possible so that it can be surgically removed.

Apart from an acoustic neuroma the differential diagnoses of causes of a unilateral or asymmetric sensorineural hearing impairment are measles, mumps, meningitis, trauma (head injury, barotrauma or surgery), asymmetric noise exposure and ototoxic antibiotics. These can all usually be fairly easily identified from the history.

There remains a large idiopathic group but it is important that before a patient is included in this group an acoustic neuroma is excluded. This can only be done by specialized audiometric tests or radiology. As such, all individuals with a unilateral sensorineural hearing impairment without an obvious cause should be referred to an otolaryngologist for screening. The incidence of acoustic neuroma in such individuals will be low, but the benefit of early diagnosis is great in terms of reduced postoperative morbidity.

■ Conclusions

- Conductive hearing impairments are often unilateral or asymmetric.
- Sensorineural unilateral or asymmetric hearing impairments are relatively uncommon but all those without an obvious cause from the history should be referred to exclude an acoustic neuroma.

Sudden hearing loss

Sudden deteriorations in hearing should be considered an otological emergency, as the diagnosis is best made by a specialist during the acute episode. Only the specialist can distinguish accurately between a conductive and a sensorineural impairment. Specialist monitoring is also important because, in the case of barotrauma, surgical management may be deemed necessary. In general, a considerable proportion (70 per cent) will recover spontaneously but it is the remaining 30 per cent who should concern us. At present there is no way of identifying who will and who will not recover, so it is necessary to see all individuals with sudden hearing loss as soon as possible.

Most sudden hearing losses are unilateral but occasionally they are bilateral. Vertigo is usually also present but may be mild.

Known causes

The aetiological factors responsible for sudden hearing loss have not all been identified. Those that are recognized can usually be identified from the history (*Table 1.3*) supplemented occasionally by clinical findings. Once all the known factors have been excluded the aetiology is a matter for conjecture.

Table 1.3 Diagnosis of sudden hearing loss

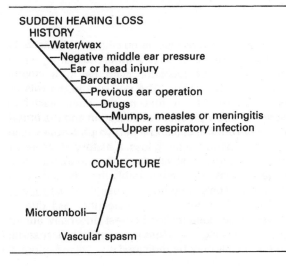

SUDDEN HEARING LOSS
HISTORY
—Water/wax
—Negative middle ear pressure
—Ear or head injury
—Barotrauma
—Previous ear operation
—Drugs
—Mumps, measles or meningitis
—Upper respiratory infection

CONJECTURE

Microemboli—

Vascular spasm

Water/wax

These are the commonest causes, singly or in combination. Bath or shower water can simply load the tympanic membrane and cause the hearing to diminish but it can usually be cleared by shaking the head. Water can also cause epithelial debris and wax to swell and block the canal. Finally, wax can be impacted against the tympanic membrane by the improper use of a cotton bud. Though it might be thought that these causes will be apparent to patients, this is not always the case.

Negative middle ear pressure/early otitis media with effusion

Many individuals will develop negative middle ear pressure because of Eustachian tube dysfunction associated with a cold. If persistent, early otitis media with effusion will develop. The diagnosis is made by the association with a cold, a history of previous episodes, the inability to auto-inflate the ear(s) and otoscopy. The hearing impairment is minimal and self-resolving.

Barotrauma

The changes in middle ear pressure associated with poor Eustachian tube function are gradual. However, it is a different matter, when there are extreme changes of pressure such as in a poorly pressurized aeroplane or when diving. The pressure in the middle ear is then grossly different from that in the inner ear. The Eustachian tube does not allow pressure equalization and the round window membrane may rupture, causing a perilymph fistula which results in a sudden sensorineural hearing loss. A history of recent air travel or diving should, therefore, always be enquired about when there is a sudden hearing loss. Almost invariably there is associated vertigo, which may not be complained of because it can be mild.

The treatment of a sudden sensorineural hearing loss due to barotrauma is admission to hospital for bedrest and daily audiometric monitoring of the hearing. If the loss is severe or progressing, surgical closure of the fistula may be indicated.

Previous ear operation

In a patient with a sudden hearing loss it is important to ascertain whether there has been a previous operation on the affected ear.

Ears in which the oval window has been opened, as in a stapedectomy, are particularly at risk of developing a perilymph fistula in the same manner as in barotrauma, but at the oval rather than the round window. In these circumstances there need be no great pressure change; a cough is all that is required to cause a break. The loss of hearing is almost always associated with vertigo and the management is surgical sealing of the oval window.

Ear and head injuries

Such injuries can cause either a sensorineural loss due to inner ear damage or a conductive hearing loss due to middle ear bleeding with or without ossicular chain disruption (page 175). A conductive impairment may particularly benefit from surgery.

Drugs

The aminoglycosides (streptomycin, kanamycin, tobramycin, gentamicin) and diuretics (especially those administered intravenously) are particularly ototoxic and as many of these drugs are excreted by the kidneys, patients with renal failure are especially at risk. Once a sufficient concentration of the drug is achieved in the perilymph the hair cells are damaged, thus producing a sensorineural hearing loss which may affect one or both ears. Monitoring of serum levels can help to reduce the incidence of ototoxicity but should a patient develop a hearing loss, tinnitus or vertigo whilst on any drug, it should be stopped immediately unless necessary for life. Thereafter, the hearing should be monitored, as the hearing loss can still progress because of selective concentration of the drug in the inner ear.

Cisplatinum is a cytotoxic drug used to treat gynaecological and head and neck tumours, which is unfortunately also ototoxic. The development of tinnitus is sometimes an alertor to developing problems.

Mumps, measles, meningitis

These three relatively common infections of childhood are recognized to cause neuritis, and the commonest single cranial nerve to be affected is the VIII nerve. Fortunately this complication is relatively rare and often on one side only. The sensorineural hearing loss often goes unrecognized at the time and there is no proven management, although steroids have been suggested. It is unlikely that subclinical mumps or measles is a common cause of sudden hearing loss but if either is suspected serial antibody titres at the time will aid the diagnosis.

Upper respiratory tract and renal infections

Sudden sensorineural hearing losses are often attributed to a recent cold or influenza. On occasions this may be the case but, considering the high incidence of upper respiratory tract infections in the population at any one time, it is not surprising that individuals with a sudden hearing loss often have such a history.

Idiopathic sensorineural causes

Having excluded the known causes from the history, the clinician is often left to conjecture the aetiology of the sudden hearing loss. The most commonly postulated factors are all vascular and it would seem highly probable that, as the inner ear is supplied by an end artery, thrombosis, microemboli or spasm can be responsible. However, unless there is evidence of such pathology in other organs, there is no way of confirming this suspicion. Vascular dilators, anticoagulants and steroids have all been suggested and tried with variable results in patients with an idiopathic loss.

■ Conclusions

- Individuals with a sudden hearing loss should be referred for a specialist opinion as soon as possible.
- The known aetiological factors are best identified from the history.
- Sudden hearing loss caused by changes in atmospheric pressure and previous surgery often benefit from early surgery.

Fluctuating hearing

Outer and middle ear causes of fluctuating hearing are more common than inner ear causes. If there is not an obvious cause in the outer ear, the differentiation can be difficult and require a specialist opinion and audiometry.

Outer ear causes

Wax and otitis externa can cause a varying hearing impairment due to varying degrees of occlusion of the external auditory canal. The diagnosis should be obvious on otoscopy.

A temporary impairment due to water immobilizing the tympanic membrane after showering, or bathing, is common.

Middle ear causes

Many people experience a feeling of fullness or dullness in their ears during or following an upper respiratory tract infection. This is caused by Eustachian tube malfunction creating a negative middle ear pressure which may be followed by a small middle ear effusion. The ears look relatively normal and the hearing impairment is so minor that it usually cannot be detected audiometrically. If the impairment is helped by auto-inflation, the diagnosis is confirmed and treatment effected.

The hearing impairment associated with chronic otitis media can also vary and is often least when the ear is actively discharging because the mucopus bridges any defect in the ossicular chain or tympanic membrane. The diagnosis should be evident on otoscopy and the management is as described elsewhere (page 29).

Inner ear causes

These are extremely rare and the mechanism is difficult to define. If the episodes of decreased hearing are associated with vertigo and there is no obvious cause, it is called Ménière's syndrome. At present there is no proven medical or surgical treatment specific to Ménière's syndrome (page 77).

■ Conclusions

• Fluctuating hearing due to wax, otitis externa and chronic otitis media are common, but perhaps the commonest cause is Eustachian tube malfunction following an upper respiratory infection.
• Fluctuating sensorineural hearing impairments are rare. Ménière's syndrome is the symptom complex of episodic vertigo with fluctuating (sensorineural) hearing.

Hearing aids for the hearing impaired

Who benefits?

Attitudes to hearing aids are changing. Previously they were thought of as a stigma of old age and senility. Now they are much more openly worn though the desire remains for small and inconspicuous aids. Anybody with a hearing impairment in one or both ears, irrespective of whether it is of a conductive, sensorineural or mixed type, would benefit at least in some circumstances from an aid. In general, the poorer a patient's hearing is the greater the benefit and the more likely they are to use an aid for longer periods of time. However the limit of benefit is reached when there is no residual hearing. Here a cochlear implant (page 64) may be of value.

Unfortunately using a hearing aid is not as simple as wearing spectacles. The latter are easy to put on, require no adjusting and are not mechanical. Hearing aids require the the mould to be put in the concha which can be difficult. Aids require to be switched on and the volume set. Mechanically they often malfunction, most frequently because of battery failure. So considerable time and effort is often required to instruct the patient how to use their aid. If this is not done its use will be poor.

How do you get an aid?

Provision systems vary throughout the world but most countries have the following alternative routes.

Via an otolaryngologist Most of those being provided with an aid will be adults with a bilateral, symmetric sensorineural hearing impairment, idiopathic in origin but age related. For them a medical opinion is probably unnecessary in the absence of other otological symptoms such as otorrhoea or vertigo. On the other hand, many patients being considered for aiding will have otological disease requiring medical or surgical management but may be symptomless apart from the impairment. The two most commonly cited conditions in this category are active chronic otitis media and acoustic neuroma. Finally, there are conditions in which, though medical intervention is not necessary, middle ear surgery is a highly beneficial alternative for alleviating a hearing impairment. The two main conditions in this category are inactive chronic otitis media and otosclerosis.

So a medical practitioner's main role is a screening one to exclude other symptoms, looking in the ears to detect chronic otitis media, carrying out tuning fork tests to detect otosclerosis (normal tympanic membrane and BC louder than AC in Rinne test) and sending for audiometry those with a unilateral or asymmetric hearing impairment to detect those requiring further investigation for acoustic neuroma.

The younger the patient the more likely they are to have a conductive as opposed to a sensorineural impairment. Correspondingly it is felt that all those under the age of 65 years should have a medical assessment whereas this will be less necessary in those over 65 years, provided they are screened by the dispenser to detect disease.

Via direct referral to an audiology department In the UK, though the issue of an NHS aid is under the supervision of a consultant otolaryngologist, the practical aspects of aid fitting and rehabilitation are delegated to audiological scientists or senior technicians. In some centres a *direct referral system* is in operation whereby a patient, referred by their general practitioner, is fitted with an aid by the audiological team without an otolaryngological assessment unless they fail certain criteria.

The following is a list of those in whom an otolaryngological opinion should be sought if not previously given.

1. Under the age of 65 years.
2. Additional otological symptoms as well as hearing impairment.
3. Abnormal otoscopy.
4. Conductive impairment of 20 dB or greater on pure-tone audiometry.
5. Asymmetric sensorineural hearing impairment.
6. Inadequate benefit from previous aid.

Via private dispensers They are bound by the same guidelines as those suggested above. The only difference with private dispensers, apart from cost, is that a patient does not need to be initially referred by a medical practitioner to get an aid. Hence, screening by private dispensers should be even more rigorous than in those directly referred to an audiology department.

Which ear(s) to fit?

Audiometry will determine the degree of impairment in each ear and whether there is asymmetry or not. In general when there is a mild or moderate impairment a monaural aid is fitted to the poorer ear. If there is a severe impairment a monaural aid is fitted to the better ear. Binaural aids are a practical proposition for all but the unilaterally impaired but there is often resistance to this idea except in the more severely disabled.

What types of aids are available?

Features common to all

Hearing aids are essentially a microphone, an adjustable amplifier powered by a battery, and an earphone. In air conduction aids the sound is delivered to the ear via a mould. In the considerably less common bone conduction aids the sound is delivered by a vibrator on the skull.

The larger the battery the greater the possible increase in volume or *gain*. The battery and mechanics can be housed in the ear mould (in-the-canal and in-the-ear aids), in a casing behind the ear (*Figure 1.26*) or in a casing worn on the body. Thus, increasingly larger batteries can be housed and the maximum gain of aids is also in this order.

All aids have an O-T-M *switch*. *O* is for *Off*. *M* is for *Microphone on*. *T* is for switching the microphone to the *Telecoil* for induction loop systems (page 68).

The *frequency* of the output of an aid can be adjusted, most simply by an H (high) and L (low) tone screw or more complicatedly by electronics. Such adjustments can be particularly useful in patients with a sensorineural impairment that is abnormally shaped on the audiogram. Thus a patient with a 'ski slope' loss at the high frequencies (*Figure 1.26*), requires minimal if any amplification at the low and the maximum tolerable amplification at the high

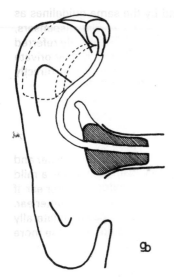

Figure 1.26 Behind-the-ear aid with standard mould

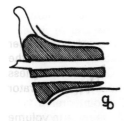

Figure 1.27 Ventilated ear mould

frequencies. The acoustical effects of aid adjustments can be measured with 'in-the-ear' microphones.

Ear moulds are cast from an impression of the outer canal and concha taken with a rapidly drying plastic material. It is possible to *vent* an ear mould (*Figure 1.27*) which makes it more comfortable to wear. Vents can also be used to modify the frequency spectrum of the output of the hearing aid complex.

Behind-the-ear aids

These are the commonest type of aid and are sufficiently powerful for all but the profoundly impaired. Unfortunately some find them difficult to position and adjust. These are the cheapest aids and in many countries are provided free by the Health Service.

In-the-ear and canal aids

These are only suitable for those with mild or moderate impairments because of the limited battery size. Because the aid is housed in a mould that has to be individually manufactured for each ear, these aids are more costly than behind-the-ear aids. Cosmetically some consider them less obvious than behind-the-ear aids but it all depends on hairstyle.

Body aids

Today these are rarely provided but they can be useful in the severely impaired that have problems with feedback. Body aids, though not troubled with feedback, suffer from clothes rub noise and are considered cosmetically unattractive because the body processor has to be connected to the ear mould by an electric wire.

Bone conduction aids

These are only necessary when there is bilateral ear canal atresia, either congenital or acquired, which prevents the use of an ear mould. They may also be advised in patients in whom the discharge from active chronic otitis media cannot be medically or surgically controlled and is aggravated by an ear mould. Conventionally the bone conductor vibrator is held on the mastoid by a head band which is both unsightly and uncomfortable. Osseointegrated titanium pegs screwed through the skin give much better attachment and can also be used to attach an ear prosthesis if the pinna is congenitally absent.

Cochlear implants

These are expensive but a serious option to consider in the profoundly or totally bilaterally impaired who get no benefit from conventional aids. Sound is converted in an external processor into electrical signals which are then fed into the implant, most frequently a multiple channel wire, that has been fed up the turns of the cochlea. This allows differential stimulation of any residual nerves along the basilar membrane and aids speech discrimination in particular. Some patients require intensive instruction in how to interpret these stimuli and unfortunately, to date, the success in children born deaf (i.e. prelingual) is marginal.

Follow-up

Once a hearing aid has been prescribed, it is essential to see the patient again to ensure that they are not having any difficulties. Many will initially have problems particularly with inserting the ear mould. This and other problems can usually all be solved but often a great deal of patience and understanding is necessary. It must be remembered that aids do not return the hearing to normal, mainly because they are amplification systems of low fidelity which boost all sounds to the same extent whether these sounds are speech or background noise. In those with a sensorineural impairment there is, in addition to a loss of volume, a loss of frequency discrimination which makes speech difficult to comprehend. For this reason, individuals with a conductive impairment benefit more from an aid than those with a comparable sensorineural impairment. Individual patients will also differ in how much benefit they get from an aid and many will find some circumstances where it is more of a hindrance than a help.

Inability to insert the ear mould

It is astonishing how many patients cannot insert the ear mould because they don't know which way it goes in. Even more have difficulty inserting the antihelical part (*Figure 1.28*) which can lead to non-use because of discomfort and feedback (*see below*). So at the return visit every recipient should demonstrate that they can insert the mould correctly, switch the aid on and control the volume. Sometimes the shape of the mould will need modification to make it easier to insert.

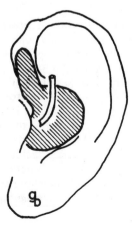

Figure 1.28 Incorrectly inserted ear mould

Feedback

Feedback is the screeching sound produced by the microphone picking up and amplifying the sound that it is putting out. The commonest cause for feedback is a poorly fitting mould, either because the mould itself is poorly made or because the patient has not put it in correctly. Moulds deteriorate and the patient's ear and canal change with time so renewal of ear moulds is frequently necessary. This is especially important with high powered aids as feedback is more of a problem with this type of aid.

Too noisy

Naturally, if one has not heard traffic and other background noise for some time, the cerebral processes which normally exclude these from consciousness have to be relearned. In addition, many individuals have to be reminded that the volume has to be adjusted in different situations.

Can't be bothered

Adaptation to an aid requires time and perseverance. Many of the elderly do not exhibit the latter and in them it is often the relatives that want to be heard rather than the patient who wants to hear. In these circumstances counselling the relatives rather than giving an aid is a sensible alternative.

Aid broken or not working

First ensure that the mould is not blocked with wax; it needs frequent cleaning with soap and water and occasionally with a nailbrush. Next make sure the parts of the aid are properly connected and that the tubing is not twisted. Switch the aid on. If there is no feedback at full volume, the battery is likely to be flat.

■ Conclusions

• As a hearing impairment may be the presenting symptom of ear disease, all patients should be screened for these before being fitted with an aid.

- Otolaryngologists are particularly adept at screening because of their skill in otoscopy.
- Active chronic otitis media is best detected by skilled otoscopy and need not be associated with otorrhoea.
- Patients with a unilateral or asymmetric sensorineural impairment should be screened for an acoustic neuroma.
- Patients with a conductive impairment can benefit from middle ear surgery for otosclerosis or chronic otitis media. Where appropriate this should be discussed as an alternative to an aid.
- The majority of aids are provided to the elderly with idiopathic, bilateral sensorineural impairments.
- Hearing aids can be of considerable benefit and nothing is lost by trying one out.
- The combination of the amount of disability, speech reading skills and motivation affects how much a patient benefits from an aid.
- Hearing aids are often not used because of insufficient explanation regarding their use.
- All patients provided with an aid should be followed-up to ensure that they can perform all the practical tasks associated with using an aid.
- Feedback can be a reason for lack of benefit but this can be overcome by ensuring that the mould fits well and is correctly inserted.
- Hearing aids and the mould need to be maintained.
- The difference between the different types of aid available is mainly a cosmetic one.

Accessory aids for the hearing impaired

The natural inclination is to fit a hearing aid and forget that for many individuals accessory aids can be of equal if not greater value.

The disability that an individual experiences with a given impairment is dependent on his lifestyle. For example, someone living alone might have the greatest difficulty listening to the television. If there are no complaining neighbours the volume is just turned-up, but if there are it might be better to suggest a television head-set rather than a hearing aid.

There are a wide variety of accessory aids available on the commercial market but they can be categorized into three types according to usage:

With a television
With a telephone
Alerting devices

   In Britain at present, these aids are not available from the National Health Service, but in certain circumstances financial aid can be given through the local Social Services Department.

Induction loops

Some but not all accessory aids use an induction loop. This is a circuit of wire into which the sound is passed electrically. This will set up, by induction, a similar electrical signal within a coil which is in the hearing aid. This is switched on by setting the hearing aid to the 'T' (telecoil) position. A loop system has the advantages of allowing the user to move around unattached to a wire and of excluding background sounds which may otherwise be troublesome. Their main disadvantage is that they pick up other electrical sounds. Loop systems can be fitted in public halls, theatres and churches as well as being used with television and the telephone.

Television aids

These can be particularly useful, especially when there are other individuals in the room who do not appreciate a loud television set. Most sets have a socket for these aids but if not they can usually be attached by a television engineer.

   There are two alternative types of aid. The first is where there is a direct output to headphones or to an ear mould. The second type uses an induction loop system; the most popular model has a loop of wire from the television in a cushion which is placed on the seat where the user sits to watch the television.

Telephone aids

The two main methods of amplification are by increasing the volume on the handset or by using a loop system. The handset can have a volume control built into it but this restricts the user to such phones. Alternatively, an amplifier can be carried around and fitted over any handset. To use the telecoil in a patient's aid requires the phone to be fitted with an induction coil. Many public telephones are now so fitted.

Alerting devices

Hard of hearing individuals are often concerned that they cannot hear the telephone or door bell. There are several solutions. The first is to change the position of the bell to a more suitable location, such as from the hall to the sitting room. The second is to get a louder bell and preferably one with a low frequency output, as most individuals with a hearing impairment are particularly affected at the higher frequencies. Flashing lights are only necessary for the profoundly hard of hearing. The final, very effective alternative, is to buy a 'wee dug' (small dog).

■ Conclusions

- Though a hearing aid will be the mainstay of management for most hearing impaired individuals, accessory aids have a considerable additional role.
- This applies particularly to the more severely impaired.
- Telephone amplification devices and loop systems in public places are the most popular forms of accessory aid.
- It is important in any individual case to take into account what difficulties he or she is having before coming to a decision as to the type of aid.

Ear syringing

When examining the ear, the view of the tympanic membrane will often be obstructed by wax. If the patient has otological symptoms the wax has to be removed as conductive pathologies are mainly diagnosed by otoscopy. If the patient has no symptoms the wax does not need to be removed. On the other hand pus and/or debris has always to be removed both to manage the condition and for diagnosis. Pus can be mopped away but it is often quicker to syringe it out.

The method of syringing is the same, irrespective of what is being removed, but, for clarity, the removal of wax will be described. If the wax is soft, it can be syringed out immediately but if impacted it requires softening. This can take several days, and may make the obstructive symptoms temporarily worse. Expensive proprietary wax softeners are not necessary, and can act as skin irritants. Sodium bicarbonate ear drops BPC are as effective and cheaper, and there is nothing wrong with olive or almond oil.

In syringing, the object is to syringe water past the wax up to the drum where it will be outwardly displaced, bringing the wax with it. Waterproof drapes are essential for the patient and for inexperienced operators. Whether the syringe is made of metal, plastic or rubber is irrelevant provided it has a blunt tip to avoid traumatizing the canal. The syringe is filled with tap water at body temperature – higher or lower temperatures can cause vertigo due to an unwanted caloric response. The canal is first straightened by pulling the pinna posterosuperiorly, and the water is directed against the posterosuperior canal wall, where there is usually a gap between it and the wax. Progress should be checked regularly by direct inspection and after completion the canal must be dried with cotton buds. Thereafter, the ear must be inspected. Gross damage is uncommon but there is usually temporary hyperaemia of the drum and canal due to the syringing.

As stated earlier syringing is one of the best methods for clearing pus and debris from the external canal as well as from mastoid cavities. The presence of infection is not a contraindication, as the middle ear is already infected. The only relative contraindication to syringing is an ear with known inactive chronic otitis media and a perforation. Even here, the chance of introducing infection is minimal if an aseptic technique is adopted and meticulous mopping performed thereafter.

■ Conclusions

- Large amounts of soft wax or pus and debris are probably most easily removed by syringing, especially by the inexperienced operator.
- Small amounts of wax are probably removed quicker with a cotton bud under direct vision.
- Impacted hard wax can be softened with olive oil, almond oil or sodium bicarbonate ear drops BPC before syringing. Alternatively, wax may be loosened under direct vision with a probe.

- The presence of infection is not a contraindication to syringing.
- Similarly, perforation of the tympanic membrane is not a contra-indication to syringing.
- The ear should always be dried and examined after syringing.

Noises in the ear (tinnitus)

Tinnitus can be a very alarming symptom, some patients consider-ing it to be the first sign of mental illness. Certainly, if the noises speak to them, they are probably correct, but otherwise patients can be reassured that it is a relatively common symptom and not a portent of mental illness, strokes or intracranial tumours.

There are two types of tinnitus. The first is otological (subjective) tinnitus, which only the patient can hear, and is usually ascribed to cochlear malfunction. This type of tinnitus is common, affecting at some time or other about 15 per cent of the population. Thankfully, the vast majority of patients are not troubled by it. The second type is transmitted tinnitus, which sometimes the doctor can hear, and is usually caused by an abnormal arterial blood flow. This type is comparatively rare and, as it usually has a beating quality, can be identified by asking the question 'Does the noise beat?'

Otological or subjective tinnitus

Otological tinnitus is often likened to a high pitched hiss or running water and is not usually pulsatile. The severity of the tinnitus can vary from day to day, but it is most often noticed in quiet surroundings and hence can be particularly troublesome in the evening when it is quiet or when the patient is trying to sleep.

This tinnitus is normally associated with a hearing impairment, although this can be so slight as not to have been noticed by the patient.

Pathophysiologically, tinnitus is considered to be an inappropriate discharge from damaged hair cells or acoustic nerve fibres, but as tinnitus is just as common in conductive as in sensorineural hearing impairments, this is not the only answer.

In a patient the main thing to assess is the degree of distress that the tinnitus is causing. The majority of individuals adjust well to their tinnitus and need no management apart from reassurance. On the other hand, there are some patients who will be depressed, but in them it is the depression that is the primary illness which requires management rather than the other way round. It is important to identify such patients as their condition requires psychological management.

Naturally, if a specific otological disease is identified which requires a hearing aid or surgery, this is recommended. The resultant improvement in hearing, by introducing previously unheard background sounds, may reduce the awareness of the tinnitus. If the otological disease does not require treatment the tinnitus can be managed in a variety of ways but unfortunately at present there are no specific anti-tinnitus drugs of proven value.

Management

1. Reassure the patient that tinnitus is not a portent of mental illness or brain disease, and that it usually becomes less troublesome with time. The majority of individuals will need nothing further.
2. Masking the tinnitus with another noise can be particularly useful in the evening or at night when the patient will be more aware of his tinnitus because there is little else to occupy his mind. Background music/speech or interstation noise from a radio or TV can be useful. To avoid disturbing a sleeping partner in bed a transistor radio can be put under the pillow.
3. Tinnitus maskers look like an ear-level or in-the-canal hearing aid but produce a background noise which many patients find to be of considerable psychological support.
4. Tranquillizers or antidepressants may be prescribed but only where considered relevant.
5. Night sedation can be prescribed.

Transmitted tinnitus

In the majority of patients with transmitted tinnitus there is a beating quality to the sound. The source can sometimes be elicited by listening over the neck for carotid artery bruits or transmitted murmurs from the heart. The skull can be listened over for an arteriovenous fistula and the ear can be looked into for a glomus jugulare tumour. This can often been as a bluish pulsation behind the tympanic membrane and can be associated with cranial nerve palsies (particularly IX, X, XI and XII) due to compression by the tumour as they pass through the skull foramina.

■ Conclusions

- Tinnitus is a common symptom.
- It is usually associated with a hearing impairment, either conductive or sensorineural.
- The hearing impairment should be managed on its own account as improving the hearing can introduce previously unheard background noise which masks the tinnitus.
- The majority of patients will learn to accept the tinnitus if reassured that it is not a portent of serious disease.
- Many find the use of background noise/music in the evening or when trying to get to sleep a useful distraction.
- A tinnitus masker is an alternative source of distracting noise.
- Some patients who are depressed complain vociferously about their tinnitus. In them antidepressant medication is indicated.
- Transmitted tinnitus from a vascular abnormality is relatively uncommon and the source may be detected by auscultation.

Disequilibrium

Most clinicians feel uncomfortable when faced with a patient with balance problems. This is partly because investigations are usually of minimal benefit in arriving at a diagnosis, making the clinician rely heavily on clinical judgement. Indeed, in the majority of individuals, no definite diagnosis will be made. Fortunately, this is not too important as the management is the same for most – reassurance that the disability will lessen with time and, if considered necessary, the prescription of one of various sedatives.

Applied neurophysiology

The clinician's first task is to elucidate the symptoms and decide the most appropriate syndrome complex the patient has. This will help to decide whether their origin is primarily otological, central or both. To understand this distinction a working knowledge of the neurophysiology is necessary.

The brain stem, acting as the coordinating centre, receives a sensory input from the eyes, from the limbs and from the vestibular

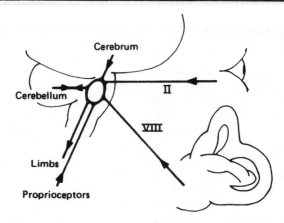

Figure 1.29 Neurophysiology of balance control

system of the two ears (*Figure 1.29*). The cerebellum coordinates body movements in response to these sensory inputs and the cerebrum exerts some overall control. Take any one of the sensory inputs away, for example by shutting the eyes, and the system will still function well. Provide a faulty or contradictory input from one and disequilibrium occurs. A common physiological cause of disequilibrium is sea sickness, when the horizon is not visually horizontal. The visual position of the waves does not tally with the input from the semicircular canals or the limbs and disequilibrium will then occur if the cerebellum cannot compensate.

Disease in any part or parts of the system can cause disequilibrium. Eye disease is not discussed further because of its rarity, and proprioceptor disease is not discussed as it should be readily identified by the associated problems of controlling the limbs.

What are the patient's symptoms and what syndrome is most likely?

In the majority of individuals with disequilibrium it is the history that enables a diagnosis to be made but this takes time and is not easy. It is far better to take time in taking the history rather than investigating the patient as investigation is seldom of great value. What actually happens during an episode of disequilibrium is the first thing to enquire about and in general the patient will complain of one of the following.

Vertigo This is the sensation of rotation or movement, either of the patient or the surroundings and is often accompanied by nausea and occasionally vomiting. Those who have drunk alcohol to excess will probably recognize the symptoms, especially the fact that the symptoms are made worse by shutting the eyes. Vertigo is most frequently a result of otological pathology, but not all otological pathology causes vertigo. The first episode of vertigo tends to be the worst and if there are any subsequent episodes these tend to be less severe because the system compensates.

Lightheadedness This symptom has no need of a description but it is important to know whether lightheadedness occurs on changing the body's position as the patient can be advised to do this more slowly. The most likely cause is postural hypotension which occurs when the body's pressure receptors are unable to respond fast enough to a change in posture, most notably on getting up from a sitting or lying posture. Typically, the patient has lightheadedness only when getting up and the effect is mitigated by getting up more slowly. Hypotensive medication for hypertension does not help postural hypotension. Any drug, in fact, can cause lightheadedness, including those prescribed for disequilibrium. This is one of the easier diagnoses to prove as the cessation of medication or changing to a different pharmacological group of drugs should relieve the symptoms.

Imbalance This typically occurs on movement, the patient often staggering to one side in particular. There are many causes for this, not least the general incoordination which goes with ageing. Most patients with imbalance usually have non-otological problems but otological disease, in the acute stage, can cause imbalance. This tends to be compensated for with time whereas central causes do not.

Blackouts/falls The patient will usually have no difficulty in deciding whether he temporarily loses consciousness, falls to the ground, or both. Such a history will rule out otological conditions as being responsible.

Having elucidated what form the disequilibrium takes, the clinician has then to decide by further questioning which symptom complex the patient is most likely to have. At this stage it is worth stating what these complexes are, particularly as clinical examination and laboratory investigation will be helpful in only a few cases.

Otological syndromes and conditions causing disequilibrium

Vestibular neuronitis

This has a typical presentation of acute, often prostrating vertigo which can take several days to settle. There are no other neurological symptoms and in particular no hearing loss or tinnitus. The aetiology is uncertain but presumed to be either viral or ischaemia of the vestibular division of the cochleo-vestibular nerve. Clinically there is usually nystagmus. In most, the system gradually compensates and there is no further trouble. If the problem continues, subsequent episodes become progressively less severe and less frequent, and will usually disappear completely after 12–18 months.

Acute labyrinthitis

This is similar to vestibular neuronitis but with the addition of loss of hearing and sometimes tinnitus. Again in most the cause is unknown. In most, trauma in this instance is a possible cause, from a head injury, ear surgery or barotrauma.

Chronic labyrinthitis

The episodes last minutes rather than days and are not grossly disabling because the system has learned to compensate. There may or may not be an associated hearing impairment or tinnitus. There are four recognized subgroups which will account for most, but not all, patients with chronic labyrinthine dysfunction.

Chronic otitis media can cause vestibular dysfunction either by irritation of the vestibular labyrinth or by erosion of the bone covering the lateral semicircular canal.

Positional vertigo is characterized by sudden, relatively short episodes of vertigo which only occur when the head is in certain positions. It occurs whether the neck is hyperextended or not and is thus differentiated from vertebrobasilar ischaemia (see below).

Acoustic neuromas are neurofibromas of the vestibular nerve which, although simple tumours, can cause death by pressing on the brain stem. It is, therefore, important to diagnose them early to enable surgical removal with as little neurological damage as possible. Acoustic neuromas have a variable presentation but almost invariably there is a unilateral hearing impairment. Disequilibrium is not common because the growth of the tumour is so slow that compensation occurs. It is important, however, to screen all patients with disequilibrium to identify whether they have a unilateral hearing impairment.

Ménière's syndrome is the symptom complex of episodic vertigo and fluctuating sensorineural hearing impairment which is usually accompanied by tinnitus and fullness in the ear(s). Like most vestibular problems, the vertigo becomes progressively less severe and frequent with time but the hearing impairment may become permanent. Ménière's syndrome is relatively rare, although the title is often erroneously ascribed to any dizzy patient. The pathological correlate is *endolymphatic hydrops*, the scala media being distended and presumably under pressure because of excess endolymph. As yet there is no proven way of diagnosing hydrops during life so the diagnosis is always presumptive. Drugs and surgery of many forms have been used with the aim of reducing the hydrops but none have proven effective. This could partly be explained by the high natural remission rate of the untreated condition. Management, until this occurs is therefore supportive with reassurance and medication (see below).

Non-otological conditions causing disequilibrium
Ageing
This is perhaps the commonest reason for imbalance and is presumed to be due to a combination of decreased blood supply and neuronal death that occurs to a varying degree as people get older. Usually the symptoms are non-specific and no clinical signs or pathology will be detected.

Transient ischaemic attacks
These are caused by short episodes of brain ischaemia. There are many suggested causes, including spasm and microemboli. The attacks occur without warning, and the patient often forgets what happened. Apart from imbalance there are almost invariably other cerebral ischaemic symptoms, such as difficulty in speaking (dysarthria), blurred vision or weakness of limbs. Unless the attack is prolonged the patient does not fall or black out. If they do the ischaemic episode is not transient and the patient is having a stroke (cerebrovascular accident).

Vertebrobasilar ischaemia

These attacks are occasioned by neck movement, especially hyper-extension. The vertebral artery is thereby compressed by an osteophytic spur in an osteo-arthritic cervical spine and transient ischaemia occurs. Disequilibrium is usually the main symptom, but loss of consciousness and other transient neurological deficits can occur. The management is prevention of neck movement either by self-control or a cervical collar.

Epileptic fits

These should present few diagnostic difficulties because of the premonition that an attack is coming, the loss of consciousness and falling with occasional injury or incontinence.

Clinical examination

Because of time constraints it is usual for the clinical examination to be modified to fit a patient's history rather than a full neuro-otological and medical examination being performed in everyone. The following examination is the minimum which should be performed in each individual to identify otological, cardiovascular and neurological disease. It is not designed to identify the actual pathology, but to identify those patients who need referral to a specialist.

Otoscopic examination

This is mainly to exclude active chronic otitis media. If suspected, referral is required to a specialist on a semiurgent basis.

Hearing assessment

Free-field voice tests (page 12) are used to identify hearing impairments and in particular unilateral impairments which may be associated with an acoustic neuroma.

Ophthalmic examination

To identify spontaneous nystagmus. Nystagmus should be assessed by asking the patient to follow with his eyes the examiner's finger moving from a central position to either side (*Figure 1.30*). Nystagmus is a repetitious slow drift of the eyes in one direction with a rapid correction back to the starting point. If the patient has

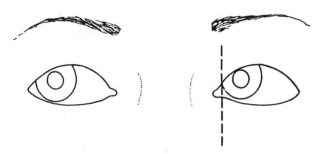

Figure 1.30 Limit of deviation of the function of the iris, the dashed line indicates the point past which the eyes should not pass while testing for nystagmus

nystagmus during a quiescent phase the pathology is likely to be central. If present during an acute episode of disequilibrium the problem is most likely otological.

The fundus should be examined to identify papilloedema which suggests increased intracranial pressure.

Cardiovascular system

This is assessed by taking the blood pressure and looking for pulse irregularities.

Nervous system

Specific screening tests are difficult to suggest. The patient's gait should identify incoordination problems of the lower limbs, particularly if he is asked to walk on a straight line or heel to toe. In Romberg's test, the patient stands with his feet together and then closes his eyes. A normal individual should be able to keep his balance. This test can be sharpened by getting the patient to stand heel to toe and/or have his arms raised with the palms up. However, even normal individuals can find this difficult for more than a short period of time.

Who to refer

It is wise for the non-specialist to refer patients for whom there is concern. The question is to whom this should be, recognizing that many patients end up being seen by several specialists.

To otologist
Chronic otitis media
Hearing impairment, especially
asymmetric
Non-resolving, peripheral-type
symptoms

To neurologist
Neurological signs
Balance/walking problems

Both will usually have access to sophisticated radiology (CT and MRI) which is perhaps the main way that intra-cranial tumours are detected. The otologist can, in addition, carry out positional testing and interpret electronystagmography and calorics.

Management

Having referred all individuals with potential otological, neurological and cardiovascular disease there will remain a large number of individuals with idiopathic disequilibrium and it is their management that is discussed.

As was mentioned earlier, it is important to elucidate the role of drugs by stopping all current medication or changing to a different pharmacological group of drugs when this is unavoidable.

In most, the mainstay of management is reassurance that the problem will resolve spontaneously. It is wise to review the patient 2 or 3 months later to ensure that this is indeed the case, and if not the patient should be referred.

In a few cases, medication will be necessary for symptomatic relief. Antihistamines, e.g. cinnarizine (Stugeron), phenothiazines, e.g. prochlorperazine (Stemetil) or a vasodilator, e.g. betahistidine (Serc) can all be tried but should not be taken for any extended period because natural resolution of symptoms usually occurs and these drugs can themselves cause disequilibrium.

Conclusions

- The diagnosis of the cause of disequilibrium is most commonly gained from the history.
- Most can be categorized as episodes of vertigo or chronic problems of balance.

- Ageing is the commonest cause of imbalance and often drugs are a contributory factor.
- Vertigo is an illusion of motion or rotation. It is most commonly vestibular in origin.
- Vertigo is often associated with other symptoms. Various commoner combinations are given syndrome titles.
- Vestibular neuronitis is a single episode of prostrating vertigo without other symptoms. Recovery may take some time.
- Vestibular labyrinthitis is the same but with an associated sensorineural hearing impairment and perhaps tinnitus.
- Positional vertigo is episodic and occurs on changing head position.
- Ménière's syndrome is episodes of vertigo with an associated, unilateral decrease in hearing and tinnitus or ear fullness.
- Chronic otitis media and acoustic neuroma are the most important diagnoses to be excluded in a patient with vertigo. The former is done by otoscopy and the latter by screening those with a unilateral or asymmetric hearing impairment.
- Once these have been excluded, a patient with recurrent episodes of vertigo can usually be reassured that compensation will occur naturally with time.
- Neurological causes for disequilibrium are comparatively rare and are usually progressive.

Facial palsy

The VII cranial or facial nerve (*Figure 1.31*) leaves the brain stem and enters the internal auditory canal of the temporal bone along with the VIII cranial (auditory) nerve. It continues through the middle ear within a bony canal and then down through the mastoid air cells before it exits into the neck through the stylomastoid foramen which is deep to the tip of the mastoid process. It then divides into several branches while running through the parotid gland, whereafter it supplies the muscles of facial expression.

Within the temporal bone it has three branches, the greater superficial petrosal nerve to the lacrimal glands of the eye, the chorda tympani to the taste buds on the anterior two-thirds of the tongue and the stapedial nerve to the stapedius muscle in the ear.

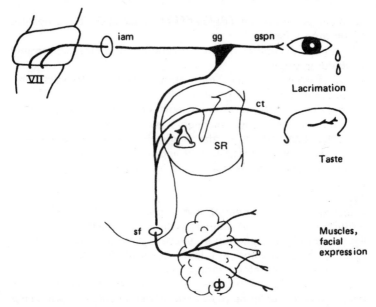

Figure 1.31 *Anatomy of the VII (facial) cranial nerve.* iam, internal auditory meatus; gg, geniculate ganglion; gspn, greater superficial petrosal nerve; ct, chorda tympani; sf, stylomastoid foramen; SR, stapedius reflex

How to arrive at a diagnosis and manage it
(see Flow Chart 5)

The cause of a facial palsy must be presumed to be in the ear or parotid until otherwise excluded. This is because disease at these sites can require treatment. In the majority of instances no definite aetiology for the facial palsy is ever identified (*Table 1.4*), but the routine assumption that this is the case inevitably means that many correctable palsies of otologic origin are left too late for the outcome to be favourable.

The facial nerve can be affected in any part of its course through the temporal bone, from the internal auditory meatus to the stylomastoid foramen. Perhaps the commonest otological pathology to affect the facial nerve is active chronic otitis media. The inflammation in the middle ear and mastoid can be such that the bone covering the facial nerve is eroded and a palsy results. The patient ought to be asked about an ear discharge, but a negative response by no means excludes active chronic otitis media as many of these patients do not complain of a discharge. A competent

FACIAL PALSY

Exclude recent trauma to head, ear and face. Exclude other neurological signs

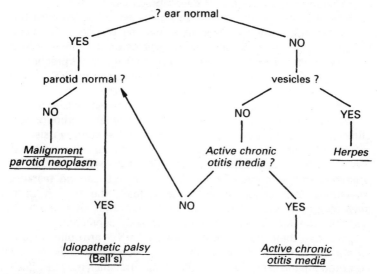

Flow Chart 5 Facial palsy

otological examination is thus essential and to do this properly all wax and debris must be removed.

Two other common otological causes of a facial palsy, temporal bone fracture and surgical trauma, are relatively easy to identify by taking a history.

Table 1.4 Commoner sites and causes of facial palsy

Site	Cause
In cerebrum, brain stem	Cerebrovascular accident (stroke)
In the temporal bone	Chronic otitis media
	Acute otitis media
	Herpes
	Head injury with fracture
	Ear surgery
Outside the temporal bone	Malignant parotid neoplasm
Unknown	Idiopathic (Bell's) palsy

If one of the above otological causes is identified an otological opinion must be sought regarding the advisability of surgical exploration, to either repair or decompress the nerve.

The remaining common cause for a palsy within the temporal bone is a virus, most often herpes. In a few the diagnosis is obvious because of the presence of herpetic vesicles on the pinna or in the external auditory canal, but in the others the diagnosis is presumptive because of a close time relationship of a generalized viral infection with the onset of the palsy. As opposed to the other otological causes of a facial palsy, the majority of virally induced palsies recover spontaneously and the management is symptomatic, although some clinicians prescribe steroids, which is somewhat controversial.

Clinically, the level of involvement of the facial nerve within the temporal bone can often be identified by testing the various branches of the nerve (*Figure 1.31*). The eye can be tested by measuring tear secretion (Schirmer's test), the branch to the stapedius muscle by provoking a stapedial reflex (tympanometry) and the branch to the tongue by testing taste sensation.

The above, then, are causes of a facial palsy that are quite obviously within the temporal bone. Of the other recognized sites the most common are the brain stem and the cerebrum which may be affected by a cerebrovascular accident (stroke). This diagnosis should be readily made because other cranial or motor nerves will almost invariably be involved (e.g. hemiparesis). When the cause of a facial palsy is above the brain stem, that is, an upper motor neuron palsy, movement of the forehead on the side of the palsy is preserved because of cross-innervation in the brain stem. The other main site for the facial nerve to be affected is once it leaves the skull, the most likely pathology being a malignant parotid tumour, but it is a misconception that malignant tumours will be obvious. Indeed if the neoplasm is in the parotid 'tail' below the angle of the jaw it can be almost impalpable. Benign parotid neoplasms do not cause facial palsies.

Management of idiopathic palsies

After exclusion of the known causes it is normal to call the palsy an idiopathic lower motor neuron or Bell's palsy and this is numerically the largest single group of palsies. Eventually, as a result of research, the aetiology of a proportion will perhaps be found to be viral, another proportion vascular, another proportion autoimmune and so on. In the meantime the main question is how to manage the individuals in whom no aetiological factor has been identified. Various forms of treatment have been advocated, including steroids and vasodilators, but there is little scientific evidence to support their use and they are less favoured than formerly. The majority (approximately 85 per cent) of idiopathic palsies recover completely without treatment. Almost all of the remainder recover to a reasonable extent but an unfortunate few end up with facial distortion which may require attempts at surgical correction. Various electrophysiological tests have been used to try and identify those palsies unlikely to recover but they have not gained universal acceptance because of their variability.

The main disabilities that individuals with an idiopathic facial palsy have are psychological. Once the recognized causes for a palsy have been excluded they can be reassured that it will almost certainly improve. At most any residual weakness will be slight: drooling of food out the corner of the mouth will stop, and the excess eye watering (due to non-draining of tears via the lacrimal duct because of weakness of the orbicularis oculi muscles) will lessen.

Management common to all facial palsies

The most important complications of facial palsy, whatever the aetiology, are ophthalmological. Conjunctival infection and corneal trauma can occur because of the absence of protective blinking. Partial suturing together of the outer eyelids (tarsorrhaphy) helps to overcome this and should be performed early when complications are anticipated, rather than too late when they have occurred.

■ Conclusions

- Facial palsies should be presumed to originate in the ear or the parotid until proven otherwise.
- Middle ear infection is the main otological pathology to be excluded.
- The management of this is surgical.
- The other common otological causes are temporal bone fractures and herpes virus infections.
- Various tests of the branches of the facial nerve may help determine the level of involvement within the temporal bone.
- A malignant parotid neoplasm can also cause a facial palsy.
- If no cause for the palsy is identified, it is considered an idiopathic or a Bell's palsy.
- There is no proven medical management for idiopathic palsies.
- In any palsy, eye complications are to be guarded against, especially when the palsy is complete.

The nose

Applied anatomy

The external nose consists of a bony part and a cartilaginous part which are integrated (*Figure 2.1*). The bony part consists of two nasal bones which interdigitate with the frontal bone and the frontal process of the maxillae. The cartilaginous part consists of five separate hyaline cartilages: the septal cartilage divides the nasal cavity in two and supports the paired upper lateral and lower lateral (alar) cartilages.

The function of the nose is to filter, warm and humidify the inspired air and this is achieved mainly by means of the large area of mucus secreting epithelium. Gross particles in the inspired air are caught in the hairs of the nasal vestibule. The air then flows in a well defined manner between the septum and the three turbinates on the lateral wall (*Figure 2.2*). The interior of the nose and sinuses has a highly

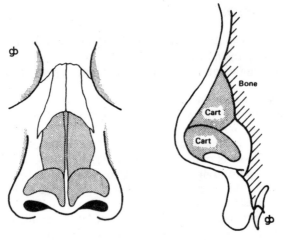

Figure 2.1 Bony and cartilaginous components of the external nose

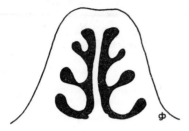

Figure 2.2 Cross section of a nasal cavity. Note the normal asymmetric nature of the septum and the unequal size of the turbinates

vascular mucosa, permanently coated by a layer of mucus which is carried by the mucosal cilia to the nasopharynx where it is either swallowed or spat up according to local culture. This mucus coating warms and humidifies the air as well as filtering out any fine dust particles. Closely integrated with the nasal cavity are the nasal sinuses which for descriptive, but not necessarily for functional, purposes are divided into the maxillary, the ethmoidal group, the frontal and sphenoid sinuses (*Figure 2.3*). These are also lined by a ciliated mucus secreting epithelium and, with the main exception of the sphenoid sinus, drain into the nose below the middle turbinate.

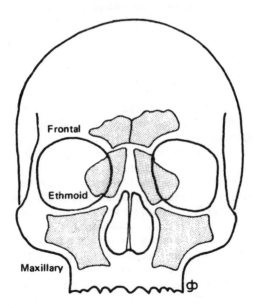

Figure 2.3 Nasal sinuses

The lacrimal duct, carrying tears from the eyes, drains below the inferior turbinate.

The nose is also the organ of smell, with the olfactory sense organs, situated in the uppermost part of the nasal cavity.

Nasal symptoms

The main nasal symptom attributable to mucosal pathology is excess mucus secretion and nasal obstruction. The nasal cavity need not actually be blocked to cause the sensation of obstruction, an alteration in the normal pattern of air flow is sufficient. As such, anatomical deformities can give the sensation of obstruction although the airway is not physically blocked. Obviously, when in addition the mucosa is oedematous, this will add to the sense of obstruction. Surprisingly, loss of the sense of smell (*anosmia*) though often present, is rarely complained of. A foul smell (*ozoena*), due to the anaerobic infection that is sometimes associated with foreign bodies and tumours, can be noticed by others and sometimes by the patient. Mucosal disease is almost invariably bilateral so unilateral symptoms should raise suspicion of other pathology, namely tumours. Because of its abundant vasculature the nasal mucosa bleeds easily (epistaxis).

Examination

Clinical examination of the nose can be extremely useful in determining pathology: the nose should always be examined externally and internally.

External examination should detect anatomical deformities of the bony and/or cartilaginous skeleton. Internal examination requires a good light and something to hold the nares open, either a hand-held nasal speculum or one mounted on an auroscope. Anterior rhinoscopy should reveal the anterior part of the septum and the inferior turbinate. In some individuals an even larger area can be visualized. Anatomical deformities, mucosal oedema and secretions are looked for. Anterior bleeding points especially on Little's area should be definable. Nasal polyps of sufficient size to cause obstructive symptoms can usually be seen, although the inexperienced often consider the turbinates to be polyps. Specialists now frequently use rigid endoscopes with the aid of topical anaesthesia to gain better views of the more inaccessible parts of the nose – in particular the osteomeatal complex where the sinuses open below the middle meatus. Posterior rhinoscopy using a postnasal mirror is infrequently performed by non-specialists but can be extremely useful in detecting adenoid hypertrophy, postnasal polyps and tumours. If there is any doubt about nasal pathology an expert opinion should be sought.

Nasal trauma

Trauma can cause damage to either the bony or the cartilaginous components of the nose (*Figure 2.1*), or to both. The bony component usually fractures, while the cartilaginous component most commonly buckes but can also fracture.

A boot, a fist, the 'close stairs' and many more innocent accidents can cause a nasal injury. The mechanism of injury is of interest but usually of minimal help in assessing the degree and type of injury. In the first few hours there will usually be generalized swelling, bruising and tenderness and at this stage clinical assessment can often be misleading. An easier assessment can usually be made 24–48 hours following the injury.

Diagnosis of extent of injury

The first question that arises is 'Has the patient broken his nose?', and here the classic signs of fracture are as applicable to the bony part of the nose as they are to any other bone in the body. There will be swelling and localized tenderness over the fracture line and some loss of function of the nose as an airway. Again, as in all fractures, there may or may not be bony displacement. Non-displaced fractures do not require manipulation, and seldom need splinting. Displaced fractures, on the other hand, do require correction both because of the visual deformity and the compromised airway. The main aim of diagnosis is, therefore, not just to define whether there has been a fracture but also to assess nasal displacement.

Essentially, displaced nasal fractures can be categorized as to whether the main direction of the force has come from the side or from the front, though, obviously, combinations can occur depending on how many times, and how, the nose has been hit.

Lateral injuries

Here, the nasal bones are fractured at their junction with the maxillae (*Figure 2.4*) and this is, therefore, the point of maximum tenderness. Displacement, if present, will be away from the side of impact and there may also be nasal broadening. In addition, the cartilaginous component will be displaced because of its attachment to the nasal bones. This will be evident by a 'C' or 'S' shaped external deformity with associated internal septal buckling. Depending on the amount of septal buckling or dislocation there may be airway obstruction or loss of nasal height. In addition, there may be a septal haematoma which merits surgical intervention in its own right because, if undrained, subsequent infection can occur which can lead to cartilage necrosis and loss of support of the nasal tip.

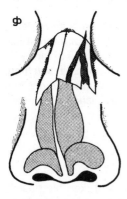

Figure 2.4 Lateral nasal fracture

While it is easy to diagnose a grossly displaced fracture it is more difficult, when dealing with a previously damaged nose, to decide whether the deformity is recent or old. In these instances, reliance must be placed on the localization of tenderness over the fracture site, and if there is doubt as to the diagnosis, little is lost by reviewing the patient 24 hours later. X-rays are notoriously unhelpful in the management of lateral injuries since they may show a fracture but do not indicate whether there is any displacement or airway obstruction which are the criteria for manipulation. Radiology is, however, helpful when other facial bones are injured in association with the nasal bones, but it is generally felt unnecessary for legal purposes provided the fact that X-rays were considered unnecessary is recorded.

Frontal injuries

Because of the inherent strength of the attachment of the nasal bones to the frontal and maxillary bones, it usually requires a strong frontal force to cause fracture. Thus, the commonest mechanism of injury is by the face being thrown against a dashboard of a car rather than by a pugilistic fist. Although the attachment of the nasal bones may be firm, the underlying bony complexes, namely the ethmoid bones, the cribriform plate and the floor of the orbit, are often involved because they are thin and, therefore, less resistant.

The clinical feature of a frontal fracture involving only the nasal bones is broadening of the nasal bridge (*Figure 2.5*). It is often difficult to distinguish such a fracture from a pure soft tissue injury

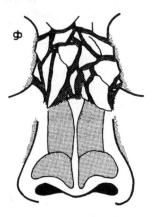

Figure 2.5 Frontal nasal fracture

due to their similar presentation. The medial palpebral ligaments are, however, attached to the bone and as these can be outwardly displaced, measurement of the intercanthal distance may be of benefit, since there are recognized normal values, as there are for the interpupillary distance. Displacement of the lacrimal sac from its groove or direct trauma to the lacrimal duct can, in addition, cause excess eye watering (*epiphora*).

Where there is sufficient frontal force, the fracture can extend to involve the cribriform plate but this often goes undetected unless made obvious by the presence of cerebrospinal fluid (CSF) rhinorrhoea. This can be difficult to recognize because a runny, bloody nose is not an uncommon symptom after any nasal fracture. The differentiation of CSF from mucus in a bloody discharge can be made by looking for a 'halo sign'. This can be seen by putting some of the secretions on a filter paper. CSF will give a halo of moisture around the blood, which mucus does not. When there is no blood in the secretions glucose can be looked for by laboratory biochemistry or Clinistix, as glucose is present in CSF but not in mucus. Cerebrospinal fluid leaking down the nasopharynx is not always apparent in the anterior nose but is often recognized by the patient complaining of a salty taste in the mouth.

Loss of the sense of smell, although invariably present in cribriform plate fractures, can also occur because the nose is blocked by oedema or blood clots. If the frontal force causing the nasal fracture has a lateral component the fracture line can run through the orbital rim of the maxillary bone, when it can usually be palpated as a 'step' on the orbital margin. On occasions, the inferior rectus muscle may be trapped, limiting upward movement of the eye, and the infra-orbital nerve may also be damaged, causing infra-orbital paraesthesia.

The possibility of the cribriform plate, the ethmoid and the maxillary bone being fractured means that radiology should be performed, although it is often unhelpful due to the thinness of the bones and because the frontal and ethmoidal sinuses will be opaque due to intrasinus bleeding. Computerized tomography can also be helpful but clinical examination is the most important factor.

Treatment

An undisplaced fracture requires no treatment apart from analgesics. A simple displaced fracture requires manipulation within ten days of injury, before reparative callus has become too firm. Under a general anaesthetic the impacted side of the fracture is outwardly displaced with forceps; thereafter the nose is repositioned by digital pressure. When the septum is grossly displaced a septoplasty at the same time will aid realignment. In some, disimpaction may be impossible and in these instances there is almost certainly an old fracture which was not previously identified. In these circumstances there is little point in continuing manipulation.

Following a successful manipulation it must be ascertained that the septum has returned to the midline and that any subperichondrial haematoma has been evacuated. Some will stabilize the mobile nose with an external plaster splint and intranasal packing. As an unsatisfactory result is common, the patient should be reviewed several weeks, and probably also 6 months, later.

For the patient with an old lateral displacement, the most satisfactory treatment is a septorhinoplasty. Frontal nasal fractures that are associated with ethmoidal or maxillary fractures usually require a combination of closed and open reduction with wiring of the fragments (page 169).

Cerebrospinal fluid rhinorrhoea merits prophylactic antibiotics to prevent ascending meningitis. The majority of leaks cease within ten days but if this does not occur surgical closure via either an extracranial or an intracranial approach, may be merited.

■ Conclusions

- Nasal fractures are mainly diagnosed on clinical grounds.
- The main clinical difficulty is distinguishing between an old and a recent fracture.
- Lateral displacement of the nose is invariably associated with septal displacement.
- Such injuries are treated by closed manipulation within 7–10 days of injury and septorhinoplasty thereafter.
- Nasal broadening of the bony bridge is caused by frontal blows and can be associated with intra-orbital and lacrimal apparatus complications or cerebrospinal fluid rhinorrhoea.
- These injuries are best managed by a combination of closed and open reduction, with bone wiring or packing.

Epistaxis

When an adult or a child presents with blood dripping from their nose, the prime aim must be to find whether the bleeding point is anterior or posterior, as the management of each is different. Anterior bleeding occurs primarily in children but also in adults. Posterior bleeding occurs solely in adults. The anterior part of the nose is easy to examine and, if an anterior bleeding site cannot be seen, by exclusion the bleeding must be posterior. Sometimes a patient presents with bilateral bleeding which can cause confusion because it is extremely rare to have bilateral bleeding points. What is happening is that blood is tracking from one side round the septum posteriorly and out the other nostril. Hence attention should be paid to the side that first bled.

Anterior bleeding

This is the commoner site in both adults and children but, because it stops in most patients with simple measures, it is considerably less troublesome than posterior bleeding. The bleeding usually comes from vessels just inside the nasal alae on Little's area on the septum (*Figure 2.6*). It has been suggested that bleeding is commoner from this site because it is the central point of the septal blood vessels but this lacks anatomical proof and is visually not evident. It is more likely that it is because crusting in this area is frequent and is accessible to a picking finger. As such, anterior bleeding is the common site in children who often pick their nose, sometimes unnoticed whilst asleep. Some adults also have this habit.

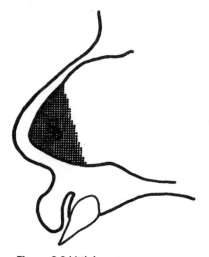

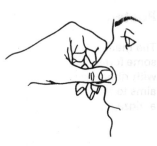

Figure 2.7 Method of compressing nose to control haemorrhage. Note position of fingers

Figure 2.6 Little's area

Anterior bleeding is simple to manage as, apart from the area being accessible to inspection, the bleeding can usually be stopped by manual compression of the anterior cartilaginous part of the nose (*Figure 2.7*). Pressure over the bony nasal bridge is commonly employed by well-meaning amateurs. 'Old wives' consider that ice packs and keys placed on strategic points around the head and neck are of benefit. All are useless manoeuvres.

If compression does not work, the next thing is to place a piece of cotton wool soaked in 1/1000 adrenaline on Little's area and compress for a further 5 minutes. When the pledget is removed, the anterior part of the nose can be inspected and the bleeding point identified. Thereafter there should be no further immediate trouble, especially in children. Their finger nails should be trimmed to prevent any further traumatic nose picking. In addition blood crusts over the bleeding points should be kept soft with white paraffin (Vaseline) to reduce the tendency to further picking and re-bleeding. If bleeding continues from an identified point, cautery can be performed using one of the numerous agents available, most commonly now silver nitrate tipped wooden sticks. To prevent skin damage, the upper lip and the nares can be wiped with white paraffin. Alternatively the agent may be applied through a metal aural speculum. Packing is usually unnecessary for an anterior bleed. If no anterior bleeding point can be identified and the bleeding continues, the bleeding point must be posterior. This occurs almost exclusively in adults with non-contractile arteriosclerotic nasal blood vessels. These patients are difficult to manage since the bleeding point is inaccessible to direct vision and to pressure.

Posterior bleeding

The management of continuing posterior epistaxis usually involves some form of tamponade. The traditional method is to pack the nose with ribbon gauze soaked in BIPP or white paraffin. This technique aims to fill the nasal cavity on the side of the bleeding by packing in a zigzag manner starting at the floor of the nostril and working

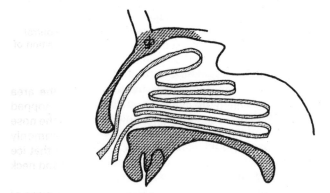

Figure 2.8 Nasal packing

cranially (*Figure 2.8*). Once in place, the pack is left for 24 to 48 hours. A modern alternative to ribbon gauze are preshaped balloon catheters which have the advantage of being easier for non-specialists to insert (*Figure 2.9*). These balloon catheters are often regarded as a form of 'instant packing' but, as their use is associated with a number of complications, they should be reserved for patients who are definitely suffering from posterior bleeding.

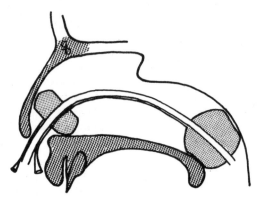

Figure 2.9 Nasal balloon catheter

If bleeding continues with a pack *in situ*, it may be necessary to try to seal off the posterior nasal aperture (choana). This can be achieved by passing a Foley urethral catheter (12 ch) along the floor of the nose and inflating the balloon once it has reached the nasopharynx (*Figure 2.10*). The proximal end is then taped to the face and the anterior and middle nose packed with ribbon gauze. The object of the pack is not to exert pressure on the bleeding point but rather to seal off the nasal cavity at both ends, by impacting the balloon in the posterior choanae and closing the anterior nares with ribbon gauze. Bleeding is then almost certain to stop as the only escape route is into the sinuses which have a finite capacity. Unfortunately, this produces large sinus blood clots which resolve slowly and are, in theory, a good culture medium. It has been recommended that prophylactic antibiotics should be given to prevent these clots becoming infected but their value is debatable. The use of packing or balloons has the disadvantage that the actual source of the bleeding is never identified or directly treated.

It is now becoming more frequent specialist practice for otolaryngologists to treat posterior epistaxis using endoscopic techniques

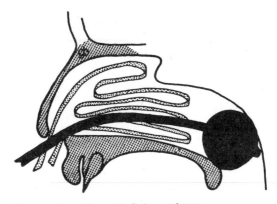

Figure 2.10 Postnasal packing with Foley catheter

which allow direct visualization and electrocautery of the bleeding point with local anaesthesia. In some patients, a general anaesthetic may be necessary. If this is unsuccessful or, if the bleeding point cannot be located, surgical ligation of the arterial supply to the nasal cavity is required. As the blood supply to the nose comes mainly from branches of the external carotid artery, this can be ligated in the neck. Alternatively, the internal maxillary which supplies the majority of the posterior nose, can be ligated via a maxillary antrum approach. The ethmoidal arteries, which are branches of the ophthalmic artery and supply the vault of the nose, can be ligated via an inner-canthal approach. See Flow Chart 6.

General consideration

If there is any doubt about management, patients with a posterior epistaxis must be admitted to hospital and an intravenous drip set up. Blood should be grouped and crossmatched, but it is usually unnecessary to transfuse except when shock is anticipated or where the blood loss is calculated, either from the volume bled or from the drop in haemoglobin level, to be at least 2 pints.

Investigation of aetiology

Once the bleeding has ceased and any packing or balloons removed, the nose should be inspected for local pathology such as tumours.

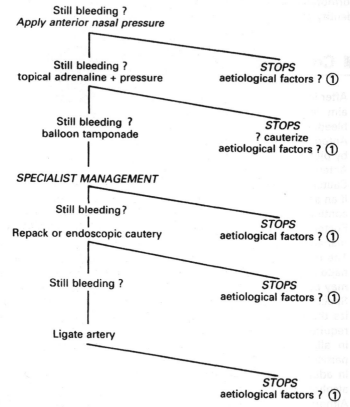

ADULT EPISTAXIS

First ensure patient does not require resuscitation or fluid replacement

Still bleeding ?
Apply anterior nasal pressure

Still bleeding ?   *STOPS*
topical adrenaline + pressure   aetiological factors ? ①

Still bleeding ?   *STOPS*
balloon tamponade   ? cauterize
                                   aetiological factors ? ①

SPECIALIST MANAGEMENT

Still bleeding?
                                   STOPS
Repack or endoscopic cautery   aetiological factors ? ①

Still bleeding ?   *STOPS*
                                   aetiological factors ? ①

Ligate artery

                                   STOPS
                                   aetiological factors ? ①

Note ① Aetiological factors to be excluded are coagulation defects
        either primary or secondary the latter being most commonly
        due to aspirin or alcohol. Local nasal factors include tumours.
        Uncontrolled hypertension should be looked for.

Flow Chart 6 Adult epistaxis

Radiology of the sinuses is of minimal value. Many patients will
have a minor bleeding tendency due to aspirin, other non-steroidal
anti-inflammatory drugs or alcohol ingestion. Epistaxis is also more
common in those with more major coagulation defects but in the
majority the diagnosis has already been made because of previous

symptoms. Hypertension must be excluded after the patient has been allowed to recover and the haemodynamics returned to normal. Epistaxis is no more common in hypertensive as opposed to normotensive individuals but the opportunity should be taken to identify previously unrecognized hypertension.

■ Conclusions

- After instituting any necessary resuscitative measures the primary aim in an individual with epistaxis is to determine whether bleeding is anterior or posterior in origin.
- Anterior bleeding is more common in children and often caused by picking crusts on Little's area on the septum.
- Anterior epistaxis is usually controlled by external nasal pressure.
- Cautery of the bleeding point is sometimes necessary.
- If an anterior bleeding point cannot be identified and the bleeding continues, the bleeding point must be posterior.
- Posterior epistaxis is commoner in adults and can be difficult to manage.
- The non-specialist management of posterior epistaxis is tamponade with balloons or gauze packing. If this fails, a post-nasal pack may be required.
- Specialist management includes endoscopy to identify and cauterize the bleeding point. If all fails, the relevant supplying artery requires ligation.
- In all, nasal tumours must be considered a possible cause, particularly if the epistaxis is recurrent.
- In adults, minor bleeding tendencies due to aspirin induced or alcohol induced platelet dysfunction should be considered.
- Although no commoner in those that bleed, the opportunity should be taken to screen for hypertension.
- Never underestimate an epistaxis, it can lead to hypovolaemic shock and death.

Blocked nose in adults

The complaint of a blocked nose without any gross symptoms such as rhinorrhoea (runny nose) can be due to a deviated nasal septum, nasal polyps or a nasal tumour. These are readily distinguished by clinical examination.

Deviated nasal septum

A deviated nasal septum is a relatively common finding on clinical examination, both externally and internally. The clinician's main difficulty is to decide whether it is actually causing airway obstruction. Complete nasal obstruction can be detected by holding a cold metal spatula below the nares and the absence of steaming up on one side suggests obstruction. When the septum has been deviated for a considerable period, particularly since childhood, there is usually a natural compensatory shrinking of the turbinate mucosa on the compromised side and a corresponding hypertrophy on the larger side (*Figure 2.11a*). This, of course, may not totally overcome the airway problem (*Figure 2.11b*).

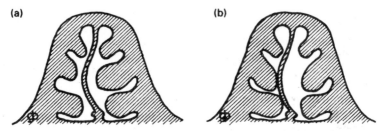

Figure 2.11 (a) Compensated septal deviation. (b) Non-compensated septal deviation

If a deviated nasal septum is considered to be the cause of airway obstruction, the only course of management is surgery. This is performed intranasally and consists of removal (submucus resection) or repositioning (septoplasty) of the deviated cartilaginous septum.

Submucus resection can only deal with internal deformaties. A septoplasty is necessary when an external deformity or anterior septal dislocation requires correction.

Nasal polyps

Simple nasal polyps are usually bilateral, although they can cause obstructive symptoms predominantly on one side. Nasal polyps arise most commonly from the ethmoidal sinuses, and their aetiology is usually unknown. Rhinorrhoea is not a common symptom and they do not bleed. There is a rare breed of nasal polyps, associated with intense asthma and aspirin sensitivity.

Examination of the nose is usually diagnostic, although the inferior turbinate is sometimes mistaken for a polyp. Differentiation is easy as polyps are insensitive to touch and are mobile.

Surgical avulsion is the usual management, but unfortunately polyps frequently recur. Intranasal steroids can help prevent this and should certainly be prescribed if recurrence is detected early. Topical steroids are sometimes used. For recurrent polyps unresponsive to topical steroids, a short course of systemic steroids can be given. Intranasal ethmoidectomy, where the ethmoids are opened up and cleared of disease endoscopically, is increasingly being practised.

Nasal tumours

Fortunately nasal tumours are relatively rare but, because of the relative size of the nasal sinuses, can be quite extensive before they present either with nasal obstruction or bleeding. Tumours are usually unilateral, hence unilateral nasal polyps should be viewed with suspicion and certainly biopsied. Sometimes, however, suspicion is only aroused by spread outside the nose to the roof of the mouth, the cheek or the orbit.

Nasal tumours are primarily managed by surgery as they are fairly resistant to radiotherapy though this may be given in addition.

■ Conclusions

- Nasal obstruction without any other gross symptoms is usually due to a deviated nasal septum, nasal polyps or a nasal tumour.
- Clinical examination should differentiate these.
- Deviated nasal septa are managed by surgery.
- Bilateral nasal polyps are usually simple and managed by avulsion.
- Unilateral or bleeding nasal polyps should be biopsied to exclude tumour.
- Nasal tumours are usually extensive when they present with nasal obstruction. Extension to the palate, cheek or orbit may be the initial presentation.
- Nasal tumours are primarily treated by surgery.

BLOCKED NOSE

A runny blocked nose or rhinitis

A runny nose (rhinorrhoea) is caused by excess mucus being produced by an inflamed nasal mucosa. The associated nasal obstruction is due to this excess mucus obstructing an airway already narrowed by oedema. Nasal mucus is clear unless the inflammation has an infective bacterial element, when the secretions will be any shade between yellow, through green to brown (*Table 2.1*).

Clear nasal discharge

A clear runny blocked nose (rhinitis) can be due to anything that causes mucosal inflammation; clinical examination usually confirms the presence of this swollen, oedematous mucosa rather than defining its cause. The aetiological factor or factors usually have to be identified from the history, as laboratory tests and radiology are of minimal value. In taking the history, the most likely cause is often arrived at by a process of exclusion, the recognized factors being viral, bacterial irritant, allergic and idiopathic (non-specific or vasomotor).

How to arrive at a presumptive diagnosis
(see Flow Chart 7)

Viral colds are the commonest cause of rhinitis but the associated prodromal symptoms, fever and other clear respiratory tract symptoms such as cough, usually make the diagnosis easy. Subsequent secondary bacterial colonization will cause the rhinorrhoea to become coloured.

Possible irritants such as dust, dry atmosphere and cigarette smoke should be considered. Although these are often the only cause of rhinitis, irritants should be assumed to be an additional factor until the other causes have been excluded.

Nasal symptoms caused by allergy can usually be identified from the history without recourse to diagnostic tests. Naturally, a patient's statement that they have an allergy needs to be probed, but it is common for the patients to have identified the allergen (provoking agent) themselves. This is particularly so when the symptoms are seasonal and can thereby be attributed to factors such as pollens. Such allergies are commonly referred to as 'hay fever' even though hay may have nothing to do with the allergy and there is seldom fever. The allergy is most usually due to pollens from the flowers of grasses, trees or flowers. Allergic symptoms are relatively specific in that as

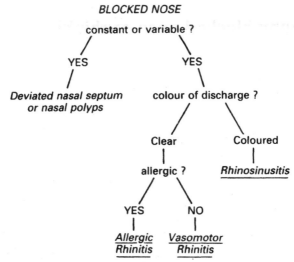

Flow Chart 7 Blocked nose

well as the nasal mucosa coming into contact with the allergen, that of the eye is also involved, so that excess watering of the eye (epiphora) is common. In addition sneezing can be marked. In childhood, nasal allergy is found in association with bronchial allergy (asthma) but they are rarely associated in adolescence and adult life. Less clear cut are allergic symptoms due to mites in house dust, animal fur or feathers, but if a definite allergy exists the patient can often relate it to certain situations such as being at home or in bed, with relief when at work or on holiday. After close questioning, symptoms that are not clearly related to a specific factor should not be labelled as allergic without further thought.

Particular care should be exercised in attributing symptoms to house dust mites, especially since many symptom-free individuals react to house dust mites on allergy testing. Allergy tests can be used to confirm the clinical impression of a specific nasal allergy but they are not often helpful as a screening procedure and are often misleading because of the high incidence (20 per cent) of positive reactions in symptom-free individuals.

If viral infections, and irritant and allergic factors can be excluded, the impressive title of 'vasomotor rhinitis' is often ascribed. There is, however, little evidence to support an autonomic imbalance and the title should be regarded as an admission that the aetiology in these cases is unknown.

Treatment of a clear nasal discharge

Irrespective of the aetiology, the treatment of a runny, blocked nose in most cases is supportive rather than curative and the same treatments tend to be given, although evidence for their efficacy has mainly come from patients being treated for seasonal rhinitis. Obviously irritant factors ought to be removed, as should any specific allergen. This is easily done if the allergy is to dog, cat or feather mites but is less easy with pollen or people.

Local steroids   Local steroids such as beclomethasone (Beconase or fluticasone (Flexonase) applied to the nasal mucosa by insufflations are of considerable symptomatic value in allergic rhinitis. Their efficacy in non-specific rhinitis is almost as marked. Systemic steroid absorption does not occur to any degree with these drugs.

Antihistamines   The main advantage of oral antihistamines against topical nasal preparations is that they can relieve eye watering that is often associated with allergic rhinitis. They are of less symptomatic benefit regarding nasal obstruction. A non-sedative (specific H-antagonist) antihistamine is probably preferable.

Vasoconstrictors   Ephedrine 0.5 per cent nasal drops BPC or similar drugs may be given for symptomatic relief during an acute episode. Its use should not, however, be prolonged because of habituation and rebound congestion when discontinued.

Desensitization   By injecting increasingly larger aliquots of the allergen, an increased tolerance is created in the allergic patient. This treatment is not now to be recommended because of the risk of fatal anaphylactic reactions.

Purulent nasal discharge

Everybody has had a purulent nasal discharge at some time or other and the symptoms probably need little description except to mention that the average patient calls it catarrh and does not differentiate between catarrh that is mucoid and catarrh that is purulent. The clinician always has to make this distinction by enquiring about the colour of the catarrh. A yellow-green or brown nasal discharge is invariably due to a bacterial infection of the mucus secreting, upper respiratory tract mucosa of the nose and nasal sinuses. Such a purulent discharge does not smell particularly offensive. If malodour is present and the discharge is unilateral, the diagnosis is most likely a foreign body. When bilateral it is most likely to be atrophic rhinitis.

The common cold virus is the common initiating factor in the production of a purulent nasal discharge. The virus affects a variable amount of the mucosa of the upper respiratory tract which thereby becomes more susceptible to bacterial infection by upper respiratory tract organisms such as *Haemophilus influenzae*, *Pneumococcus*, streptococci and staphylococci. The mucosa lining the nasal sinuses (maxillary, ethmoid, frontal and sphenoid) is almost invariably involved and contributes to the production of the purulent nasal discharge. Sinus involvement is usually, therefore, asymptomatic. If any symptom is present it is a feeling of fullness of the nose, face or cheeks rather than acute facial pain or headaches.

Acute sinusitis When facial pain is associated with sinus disease it indicates obstruction of the ostium of the affected sinus by secretions and mucosal oedema. What in effect is then present within a sinus is a non-draining abscess. The presence of facial pain, fever and tenderness over the affected sinus all suggest that this has occurred and this is clinically described as an acute sinusitis, although this term should strictly cover any acute infection of the sinus, whether the ostium is blocked or not. Acute sinusitis is a relatively rare sequela of the common cold or of chronic sinusitis (*see below*).

The purulent nasal discharge associated with a common cold rarely requires antibiotic therapy as the condition spontaneously resolves. Antibiotics are only indicated when there is gross systemic upset or when a specific individual is known to be prone to complications such as acute otitis media. Decongestive nose drops are not usually indicated, but symptomatic relief of any fever is often achieved by the use of aspirin. Steam inhalations encourage drainage of thick secretions and the addition of menthol crystals to the water gives an added sensation of relief.

Chronic sinusitis Chronic sinusitis is the likeliest diagnosis for a purulent nasal discharge. Here the symptoms are the same, with a yellow-green or brown nasal discharge, and occasionally a feeling of facial fullness rather than facial pain or headaches. In contrast to the common cold these symptoms occur frequently and can be unremitting. It is only occasionally that individuals with chronic sinusitis have pain and this usually indicates that the sinus ostium has become blocked, resulting in acute and chronic sinusitis.

When a patient presents with a recurrent purulent nasal discharge it is essential to rule out predisposing factors such as nasal polyps, grossly deviated nasal septum, adenoid hypertrophy, previous nasal surgery and dental disease extending into the maxillary sinus. If found, these usually require surgical correction. If none of these factors are present the individual has idiopathic chronic sinusitis, a condition with considerable similarities to chronic bronchitis regarding aetiology and management. The predisposing factors may be genetic, allergic and environmental, the latter most commonly being smoking and industrial pollution.

There is really no alternative diagnosis to chronic sinusitis in a patient with an anatomically normal nose and recurrent episodes of purulent nasal discharge. Radiology is not particularly helpful, except perhaps to exclude any predisposing pathology. Equally, a maxillary sinus washout will produce mucopus during an active phase and none if the patient is in a quiescent phase of the chronic sinusitis. Sinus washouts used to be the mainstay of treatment before the advent of topical steroids (Beconase) but the latter is now preferred. Septrin, erythromycin, tetracycline and ampicillin can also be prescribed when the symptoms are severe. Nasal decongestants may sometimes be of symptomatic value, along with steam and menthol inhalations. Occasionally, if topical steroids and systemic antibiotics are not effective, the maxillary sinus is explored via a Caldwell Luc approach to remove grossly diseased mucosa or antral polyps but it must be remembered that the maxillary sinus is not the only sinus that can be affected in chronic sinusitis.

■ Conclusions

- When a patient complains of catarrh, it is important to ascertain whether it is mucoid or mucopurulent.
- If mucoid, the diagnosis is rhinitis.
- If mucopurulent, the diagnosis is most likely the common cold or chronic sinusitis.
- Facial pain is uncommon in the common cold or chronic sinusitis and, if due to nasal disease at all, is suggestive of acute sinusitis.

Table 2.1 Commoner causes of rhinitis

Diagnosis	Cause
Mucoid rhinitis	Common cold
	Irritants
	Allergic rhinitis
	Non-specific (vasomotor) rhinitis
Mucopurulent rhinitis	Common cold
	Chronic sinusitis

Mouth and pharynx

Applied anatomy

The mouth and the pharynx are primarily upper alimentary structures, with respiratory tract functions taking a secondary role. Correspondingly, symptoms are related to eating rather than breathing. As well as being involved by local pathology, the mouth and pharynx can be affected by generalized alimentary disease.

Mouth anatomy

The mouth is the area where mastication and primary digestion of the food by saliva takes place. The teeth grind the food and the tongue mixes it up with saliva, which is secreted by the parotid gland opposite the second upper molar tooth and by the submandibular and sublingual glands below the tongue. Food is then formed into a bolus which is propelled backwards by the tongue. The soft palate elevates to close off the nasopharynx and the food enters the pharynx.

Pharynx anatomy

The pharynx is divided into three parts (*Figure 3.1*). The soft palate divides the nasopharynx from the oropharynx and the hypopharynx is the part below the base of the tongue down to the post-cricoid region at the inlet to the oesophagus. However, in the swallowing of food the muscles of the oro- and hypopharynx act as one entity. During swallowing, the tongue musculature pulls up the hyoid bone and, correspondingly, the larynx. This tilts the epiglottis back to protect the laryngeal inlet. The food bolus passes under the voluntary control of the pharyngeal musculature via the pyriform fossae into the postcricoid region of the oesophagus at the level of the sixth cervical vertebra. Thereafter food propulsion in the oesophagus is an autonomic process.

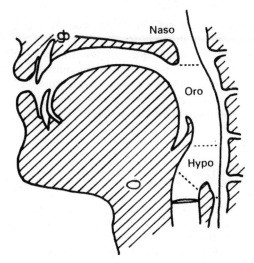

Figure 3.1 The three parts of the pharynx

At the entrance to the pharynx there are scattered aggregates of lymphoid tissue, commonly called Waldeyer's ring, which, for anatomical purposes, are grouped (*Figure 3.2*): the adenoids lie in the posterior pharyngeal wall, the tonsils lie between the anterior and posterior pillars of the fauces and the lingual tonsils are at the base of the tongue.

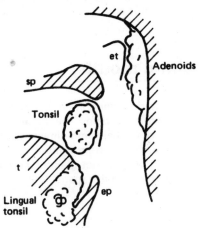

Figure 3.2 *Lymphoid tissue of the pharynx.* ep, epiglottis; et, Eustachian tube orifice, sp, soft palate; t, tongue

Pain sensation in the mouth is supplied by the V (trigeminal) cranial nerve and in the pharynx by the IX (glossopharyngeal) cranial nerve. Taste on the anterior two-thirds of the tongue is supplied by the chorda tympani via the lingual nerve and the posterior one-third by the IX cranial nerve. Tongue movement is controlled by the XII (hypoglossal) cranial nerve and the palate and pharynx by the X (vagus) cranial nerve.

Examination

The mouth and oropharynx can be readily examined provided there is good illumination and a spatula is used to retract the lips, cheeks or tongue. A handheld torch does not give either an adequate light or leave both hands free. Hence a headlight or mirror is preferable.

All areas of the mouth should be examined no matter what the oral complaint, so dentures must always be removed. Any lesion should be palpated with a finger. Indeed, if the patient considers there is 'something there', the suspicious area should be palpated even if no lesion can be identified visually.

Examination of the nasopharynx and hypopharynx requires the use of a mirror and as such is not usually within the competence of non-specialists. Correspondingly, if pathology is suspected in either of these areas, referral for clinical examination is mandatory.

Sore or painful mouth

Perhaps because of its rich innervation, the majority of oral lesions present with discomfort or pain. The patient can usually point precisely to the area of concern and clinical examination will then usually categorize the condition into one of the following types of lesion. Oral lesions that are not painful should be considered malignant until proven otherwise (page 120).

Ulcers

Small mucosal ulcers are usually painful and the diagnosis is made from experience and their site.

Aphthous ulcers recur regularly on mobile parts of the mucosa such as the cheeck and labiogingival sulci. Their treatment is topical antiseptics (chlorhexidine), astringents (zinc sulphate BPC) or hydrocortisone pellets.

Traumatic ulcers from jagged teeth or dentures are usually identified as such by the patient or by the clinician looking for a cause. Dental management is curative.

Candida yeast infections are classically covered by a white membrane which when removed reveals a raw mucosal area. Frequently there is a simple raw area under the upper denture. Patients may also have a small painful mouth with cracks at the angles; *angular cheilitis*. Patients with candidal infection are often debilitated by general disease and have been on antibiotic therapy. Treatment is with topical nystatin lozenges, cessation of antibiotics and by improved general health.

Herpetic ulcers occur on non-mobile mucosa such as the hard palate and are treated non-specifically with protective pastes (carmellose gelatin: Orabase).

Raised lesions

Fibrous traumatic polyps can be painful. They occur when the cheek mucosa is repeatedly nipped by closing teeth or dentures. Rarely do they require surgical removal.

Leukoplakia These are white plaques on the cheek or tongue mucosa caused mainly by irritants such as teeth and tobacco. If these are eliminated, the plaques will disappear. Although neoplasms can subsequently develop this is not as likely as with erythroplakia.

Erythroplakia These are red raw raised areas again related to trauma. These should always be biopsied as many are already carcinoma *in situ*.

Toothache

Dental caries are so common that it is rare, except in edentulous patients, not to be able to suggest that they have some part to play in a patient with facial pain. Dental caries are usually fairly obvious

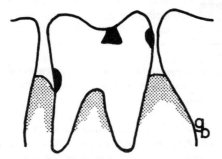

Figure 3.3 Commoner sites for dental caries

when they affect the crowns of the teeth, but they are also exceptionally common between the teeth and at the junction with the gums and this is more difficult to identify (*Figure 3.3*). Dental root abscesses are, of course, a cause of severe toothache, and here local tenderness will be pronounced and a palpable swelling of the maxilla or the jaw may be evident. The best test is to tap the appropriate tooth, which will cause discomfort.

Other

Burning mouth syndrome is a common condition which tends to progress as the day wears on. The numerous factors associated with it include denture problems, haematological deficiency, dry mouth, diabetes, thrush and psychological factors such as anxiety, depression and cancer phobia. Once vitamin deficiencies, anaemia and local pathology have been ruled out, and if the patient is obviously not psychologically imbalanced, reassurance that there is no serious disease is given.

■ Conclusions

- Painful mouth lesions are usually diagnosed by inspection.
- Treatment is usually disease specific.
- Non-painful oral lesions should raise the suspicion of cancer.

Sore throats

A sore throat is a common symptom but its true nature must always be ascertained as patients often use this term when describing other symptoms. Because of the discomfort, a true sore throat should make it difficult to swallow food or fluids and, when severe, even saliva. A feeling of dryness, excess mucus (catarrh), dry cough, altered voice and pain in the neck, are often wrongly described as a 'sore throat'

A sore throat is caused by inflammation of the pharyngeal mucosa due to either traumatic or infective agents.

Aetiology

Local trauma

Cigarette smoke is one of the commoner causes of a sore throat and the patient need not be a smoker, as pubs and discotheques frequently provide a smoky atmosphere. Indeed, sore throats are common after social events where, in addition to cigarette smoke, the pharynx receives the local trauma of alcohol.

Radiotherapy to the head and neck region almost invariably produces a dry, sore mouth and throat, both by traumatizing the mucosa and by diminishing the secretions of the salivary glands. Fortunately the effect of radiotherapy is usually temporary.

Upper respiratory tract infections

Viruses, including the common cold and adenoviruses, are the commonest infective cause of a sore throat. They affect a varying proportion of the upper respiratory mucosa, which extends from the anterior nares into the sinuses, back to the nasopharynx, up the Eustachian tubes to the middle ear, down to the oropharynx and over the tonsils, down the hypopharynx into the larynx, over the vocal cords, down the trachea into the major bronchi and eventually to the bronchioles (*Figure 3.4*). Symptoms of infection of this mucosa vary, depending on the area that is involved, but there may be any combination of the following: runny nose (coryza), sneezing, runny eyes (due to oedema of the nasolacrimal duct), dullness of hearing (due to retention of middle ear secretions by Eustachian tube oedema), sore throat, hoarse voice and a dry or mucoid cough.

If a patient with a sore throat is fevered this suggests an infective cause, and if, in addition, there are symptoms suggesting that the

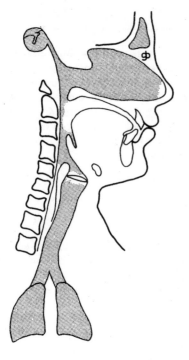

Figure 3.4 Extent of upper respiratory tract mucosa. Shaded area represents distribution of upper respiratory tract, ciliated mucus secreting mucosa

ear, nose, voice or chest are affected, then the infection is more likely to be viral than bacterial.

Secondary bacterial infection can of course occur, and this is recognized by the watery mucoid secretion becoming mucopurulent. Thus the spit or the nasal or the postnasal discharge becomes yellowy-green.

Following birth, the individual gradually becomes immunocompetent over many years. This requires repeated exposure to viruses and bacteria, the main point of entry being the upper alimentary and respiratory tract mucosa. It is natural, therefore, that in normal children there should be hypertrophy of all the lymph gland tissue in this area. This includes the tonsils, adenoids and cervical lymph nodes. Indeed it could be suggested that in children, non-enlargement of any of these is pathological.

Acute tonsillitis In acute tonsillitis, bacteria, mostly beta-haemolytic streptococci, infect the tonsil, primarily in the tonsillar crypts.

Almost invariably there is systemic upset with fever and difficulty in swallowing. The natural course is spontaneous resolution within 10 days but this can be shortened to 2–3 days if an appropriate antibiotic (penicillin) is taken. The infection does not 'go' to the chest, nose or stomach but the cervical lymph nodes become enlarged and tender.

Quinsy Occasionally an abscess (quinsy) forms in one of the tonsils and this is suspected if the patient finds the mouth difficult to open because of reflex, masseteric muscle spasm (trismus). In the early stages an abscess may be treated with antibiotics but there is the danger of a chronic septic mass resulting because of inadequate dosage. Surgical drainage at that time allows the symptoms to subside rapidly. There are different ways of doing this under local anaesthetic. The quickest and least potentially damaging is aspiration with a wide bore needle on a syringe. More conventionally a stab incision with a scalpel can be made. If these fail the presence of an abscess can be confirmed by ultrasound and then tonsillectomy under a general anaesthetic is an alternative means of drainage.

It is considered advisable, if the patient has had trouble with recurrent tonsillitis in the past, that once a quinsy has subsided tonsillectomy should be arranged for a later date. In others it is probably not indicated.

Not all children develop attacks of acute tonsillitis but in those that do the most common age of onset is 4–6 years. For an individual child, the age of onset may be different but in almost all, natural immunity develops over two to three years and the frequency of attacks then diminishes.

Differential diagnosis of a sore throat

As the majority of children do not smoke, the main difficulty is in differentiating between viral and bacterial infections. Both conditions produce fever and tender lymph glands in the neck. The diagnosis in the acute stage rests, therefore, on the presence or absence of other associated symptoms and the clinical assessment of the extent of the inflammation. Viral infections are usually associated with additional upper respiratory symptoms such as a runny nose, sneezing, watery eyes, cough or hoarse voice, whereas acute tonsillitis is not. In viral infections the majority of the mucosa of the upper respiratory tract will be involved and if any abnormality is detected at all it will be a general hyperaemia and increased irritability of the throat when it is being examined. In many instances no real abnormality will be detected. On the other hand, in acute tonsillitis the inflammation should be obvious and centred around the tonsils which will be swollen, inflamed and oedematous. On occasions 'pus' may be seen coming from a tonsillar crypt but this has to be distinguished from retained food in the crypts. If the diagnosis is acute tonsillitis and the symptoms merit antibiotic therapy, rapid improvement in the signs and symptoms should occur within 24–48 hours. If this does not occur then either the infection is viral or the possibility there is a *quinsy* should be considered.

In adolescents and adults acute tonsillitis is less common and the diagnosis rests similarly on the above criteria. An additional differential diagnosis in this age group is infectious mononucleosis (glandular fever) in which there is usually lymph node hypertrophy out of all proportion to the extent of inflammation. This hypertrophy need not be confined to the cervical lymph nodes but can also involve any part of the reticuloendothelial system including the liver and spleen.

In all patients, when they do not have a sore throat, clinical examination of the pharynx and tonsils is valueless. This is in contradistinction to the acute situation where it is diagnostic. There is no normal size for tonsils and apparent enlargement is not an indication of past infections so that the diagnosis must be arrived at on the basis of a full history, or by seeing the patient during an acute attack.

When infectious mononucleosis is suspected, the results of a differential white cell count, blood film and monospot tests will be of value. Bacterial culture of pharyngeal or tonsillar swabs has little merit in either the acute or chronic situation as differentiation from the normal commensal flora is virtually impossible. However, in some instances, serial serological tests for viral antibodies may be of value.

Treatment of a sore throat

Treatment is usually supportive until spontaneous resolution occurs, the essence being, especially in children, to ensure that an adequate fluid intake is maintained, taking into account the increased requirements due to fever. Otherwise the patients can eat and drink what they like. In adults, aspirin taken as a gargle and then swallowed, often alleviates the discomfort by having both a topical and systemic effect. In children, aspirin is contraindicated because of the risk of Reye's syndrome (encephalopathy and liver failure). Paracetamol elixir is to be preferred for those under the age of 12 years. In viral infections antibiotics have no part to play unless secondary bacterial infection causes serious consequences, e.g. acute otitis media, and even then their role is in doubt. Antibiotics have no prophylactic role in preventing such complications.

In acute tonsillitis, antibiotics should not be routinely prescribed but they may be of value if the systemic upset is severe. In the presence of repeated attacks of acute tonsillitis, the question will inevitably be raised, often by the parents, as to whether tonsillectomy would be of value. Unfortunately, tonsillectomy is one of the mainstays of private practice and this has tended to obscure the real indications for tonsillectomy and the attendant dangers. Controlled clinical trials of tonsillectomy have shown that the benefit is evident for only a couple of years because of the natural tendency for the frequency of attacks to diminish spontaneously. This natural resolution is confirmed in hospitals where there is a long waiting list for tonsillectomy. When eventually admitted the children are often symptomatically improved and in many the indications for surgery are no longer present. Although low, there is a mortality from surgery which is higher than the mortality from drug reactions to penicillin. The operation is inevitably haemorrhagic and there are psychological problems associated with admission of young children to hospital. The operation is of no value in the treatment of colds, coughs, viral upper respiratory infections or in the prevention of bacterial endocarditis and nephritis. The operation also has a 10 per cent failure rate because of tonsil remnants being left.

It might appear from the above that there are relatively few indications for surgery. It is, however, a balance of judgement regarding the incapacity caused in any particular patient by the recurrent tonsillitis against the disadvantages of surgery. Inevitably the frequency and severity of the attacks must be considered and the balance struck will be different for various surgeons, favouring operation when there has been an abscess (quinsy), against it because of the potential of creating speech problems in those with a cleft palate or a bifid uvula, and contraindicated in those with a bleeding tendency. In the absence of palatal abnormalities, this balance is not altered by any clinical finding in the quiescent phase. There is no normal size for tonsils and examination of them does not help confirm the frequency or severity of the symptoms. This is contrary to the acute situation when examination is extremely helpful in coming to a diagnosis.

It is now recognized that tonsillectomy and adenoidectomy should be considered as two separate operations each having different indications. Adenoidectomy is consequently discussed elsewhere.

The tonsils will usually be removed under a general anaesthetic by dissection which allows any bleeding points to be tied. Guillotine tonsillectomy is now rarely performed.

■ Conclusions

- Viruses are the commonest infective cause of a sore throat.
- Bacterial infections, in the form of acute tonsillitis are correspondingly relatively uncommon.
- Smoking, itself a common cause, helps neither.
- Viral infections are usually associated with nasal or bronchial symptoms (runny, blocked nose, cough, etc.).
- Acute tonsillitis is not associated with nasal or bronchial symptoms.
- Both viral and bacterial infections can be associated with fever and lymphadenopathy.
- Clinical examination in the acute stage will readily diagnose tonsillitis as the inflammation will be localized to the tonsils.
- Clinical examination in a quiescent phase is of minimal value in assessing the aetiology of recurrent sore throats.
- A sore throat is managed symptomatically with analgesics and gargles. Antibiotics should not be used routinely.
- Antibiotics have no influence on viral infections but can shorten the course of, but not prevent, acute tonsillitis.
- Recurrent viral infections, colds, runny noses, are not helped by tonsillectomy.
- Recurrent episodes of acute tonsillitis usually stop recurring.
- Tonsillectomy can reduce the frequency of attacks of acute tonsillitis during the two years it takes on average until natural immunity develops.
- A previous quinsy is by no means a definite indication for tonsillectomy.
- Tonsillectomy has a mortality, morbidity and failure rate.

Dysphagia

Technically, the term dysphagia means difficulty in eating but by common usage its use is restricted to describing the symptom of difficulty in swallowing rather than the whole range of the problems of eating.

Symptoms

Because of the relative size of the mouth and pharynx, lesions in these regions have to be very gross before there is actual obstruction to the passage of food. Lesions in the mouth and pharynx usually cause the sensation of 'something being there'. Alternatively, there can be difficulty in getting food over but once the food is over there is no further difficulty. This is in contradistinction to diseases of the oesophagus where the lumen is relatively narrow and even small lesions can cause partial obstruction. The symptoms of difficulty in eating and getting it over usually, therefore, arise from diseases of the mouth and pharynx. Difficulty in swallowing usually arises from disease in the oesophagus. In these notes it is with the mouth and the pharynx that we are particularly concerned.

History

In taking the history, it is important to assess the symptoms in detail rather than simply accepting statements such as 'rawness of the throat'. The duration and periodicity of the symptoms are obviously important but their reliability is open to question. It is also unlikely that patients with disease in the mouth and pharynx will have lost much weight unless eating is actually painful, which is uncommon. If there has been loss of weight the systemic effects of disease such as carcinoma should be suspected.

Clinical examination

The clinical examination is the crux of diagnosis in the mouth and oropharynx. In the mouth, radiology has little place except in assessing bony involvement of the mandible or the maxilla. In the pharynx, clinical examination is the single most reliable procedure but when a mirror has to be used, as in viewing the hypopharynx, its reliability is less certain. Where assessment of the hypopharynx is uncertain it is better to perform endoscopy under general or local anaesthesia, rather than on radiology. Lateral X-rays of the neck only show up gross mucosal lesions and some foreign bodies, and the main role of a barium swallow is in the diagnosis of muscular incoordination and pharyngeal pouches. The following is a list of areas which if examined during the clinical examination, will allow the clinician to arrive at a diagnosis in the majority of individuals. The list is by no means comprehensive and it is up to the clinician in each individual case to use his judgement to decide whether further areas, such as the abdomen, require examination.

Lips and oral mucosa

Examination of the lips and oral mucosa is the first opportunity to assess the alimentary tract. The lips themselves may be pale suggesting an anaemia, due to iron, folate or vitamin B_{12} deficiency. In these the whole alimentary tract mucosa is affected causing is to be dry and giving a sensation of food sticking. In many who do not wear dentures the mouth may be contracted in circumference and the angles may be cracked – *angular cheilitis* – due to candidal infection.

Eating may be difficult due to painful, mucosal ulcers (page 110). The commonest causes are recurrent aphthous ulcers and traumatic ulcers from broken teeth or rough, loose fitting dentures. It is usually easy to diagnose candidal fungal infections by their whitish covering membrane which when removed will reveal a raw area. Such infections are more frequent in debilitated patients on antibiotic therapy.

Teeth

Dental problems are the most common cause of difficulty in eating, particularly in the lower socio-economic groups. Thirty-seven per cent of the population over the age of 16 are edentulous and long-term wearing of dentures is associated with atrophy of the maxilla and the mandible, particularly the latter. With advancing years denture fitting and retention becomes a problem and is one of the reasons why a large number do not wear their dentures. Obviously, for them and for those whose dentures are loose or malfitting, eating is more difficult.

In patients with teeth, many of them are often carious and this chronic infection can predispose towards recurrent oropharyngitis. If a large proportion of the teeth have been removed, the normal apposition of the mandible and maxilla is lost, putting strain on the temporomandibular joint. This causes pain in the joint, often complained of as pain in the ear, and difficulty in eating.

The finding of dental problems does not, of course, exclude other pathologies and these must be rigorously sought before attending to the dental problems.

Tongue and oral mucosa

Carcinomas of the tongue and oral mucosa are, unfortunately, often of considerable size before being clinically detected. This is because the site of origin is frequently in silent areas such as the bucco-alveolar and the alveolar-glossal sulci. The exclusion of oral carcinoma requires a rigorous inspection of all the areas within the mouth when difficulty in eating is complained of. As mentioned above this necessitates a good light and the use of spatulae so that the cheek and the tongue can be retracted in the various directions to enable the so-called 'silent areas' to be inspected. Finger palpation can also be extremely helpful. If there are any suspicious areas a specialist opinion should be sought. Poor dentition, high alcohol ingestion and smoking are common aetiological factors in oral carcinoma so clinicians should be particularly alert in such patients.

When small, oral carcinomas are usually managed by surgery or radiotherapy and when large by surgery with reconstruction.

Oropharynx

Recurrent pharyngitis is probably the commonest cause of difficulty in eating. In the majority of patients it is of an episodic nature but in some the symptoms can be chronic. In the majority, viral infections are responsible and as viruses affect all types rather than specific areas the whole of the mucosa of the pharynx is usually involved. During an acute attack of pharyngitis the clinical signs are often minimal. In some there will be a slight increase in redness and in the gag reflex but in others the pharynx may appear entirely normal. When the symptoms are acute, discomfort is fairly predominant. In the chronic situation, this is less so and difficulty in getting food over is more often complained of. Clinical examination in the chronic situation is even more unreliable. Irritant factors, such as smoking or dust, should be identified from the history and avoiding them often improves the symptoms, helping to confirm the clinical diagnosis.

'Big' tonsils are never as big as they might appear clinically, since the act of opening the mouth and saying 'Ah' lifts the soft palate and hence elevates the tonsils into a more prominent position. The tonsils then, although often appearing to occlude the oropharynx, seldom do so and correspondingly rarely cause dysphagia by dint of their size. They will, however, cause dysphagia if they become inflamed.

In the oropharynx the tonsils are the most frequent site for carcinoma. As only one tonsil is usually involved, any degree of asymmetry of tonsil size in someone who complains of 'something there', or food sticking is an indication for biopsy. Histologically, carcinomas are either squamous carcinomas or lymphomas.

Hypopharynx

There are three relatively common, non-neoplastic conditions that affect the hypopharynx.

Pharyngeal pouches are relatively rare and are thought to be due to secondary swallow in a megapharynx along with a weakness in the pharyngeal muscle layers through which the mucosa herniates. The hernia gradually extends into the neck and causes a relative obstruction because of external pressure on the pharyngeal wall from retained food within the pouch. As the inlet to the pouch cannot usually be seen either by direct or indirect examination the diagnosis rests on radiological visualization of swallowed barium within the pouch. Pouches are usually surgically excised via the neck or alternatively can be opened into the main lumen by endoscopic diathermy or laser division.

Muscular incoordination is an increasingly recognized entity and can be simply local muscular incoordination or part of generalized neurological disease. When part of general disease, such as motor neuron disease or pseudobulbar palsy, there is often overflow into the laryngeal inlet during eating with coughing and aspiration. Local muscular incoordination is akin to inability to squeeze a tube of toothpaste consistently along its length to produce a flow. Muscular incoordination is diagnosed by seeing an abnormal peristaltic pattern on a video tape recording of a barium swallow, and is difficult to manage, there being no specific therapy.

Generalized neurological disease such as motor neuron disease or pseudobulbar palsy is usually much more severe and usually fatal. Indirect laryngoscopy often reveals a lax, immobile pharynx with pooling of saliva in the hypopharynx. Overflow into the larynx and lungs readily occurs with coughing and aspiration pneumonia. Management is extremely disappointing, myotomy and feeding gastrostomy being palliative rather than curative procedures.

Neoplasms can enlarge to considerable size, for example in the pyriform fossae, until they present with symptoms which may be laryngeal rather than alimentary. The exceptions are postcricoid carcinomas which technically are in the pharynx but anatomically and physiologically are more part of the oesophagus.

Oesophagus

The main symptom that would suggest oesophageal pathology is actual obstruction to swallowing. Pathology most commonly occurs in the upper third in the postcricoid region and in the lower third at the oesophageal gastric junction. Lesions in the lower third are usually the province of the thoracic or gastro-enterological surgeon and are not dealt with here but it is important to remember endoscopy is almost always required to exclude oesophageal malignancy.

Postcricoid lesions have an association with iron deficiency anaemia whose mucosal effects have been mentioned earlier and were initially described by ENT surgeons (Paterson and Brown-Kelly). Such anaemias are more common in females and in a certain percentage of them a web develops in the mucosa in the postcricoid region. This causes a holdup of food and difficulty in swallowing. In an even smaller proportion of these individuals a postcricoid carcinoma develops. Webs and postcricoid carcinomas do, of course, occur in the absence of anaemia.

Webs are stretched endoscopically and any anaemia treated appropriately. Carcinomas have usually involved the larynx by the time they are diagnosed, so pharyngolaryngectomy with reconstruction is the management of choice for cure.

Management

From the above it will be fairly obvious that a clinical examination supplemented by a barium swallow and haematological screen will diagnose the majority of pathologies, each of which has its own specific management. In general, small carcinomas are treated with radiotherapy giving a reasonable cure rate, but unfortunately by the

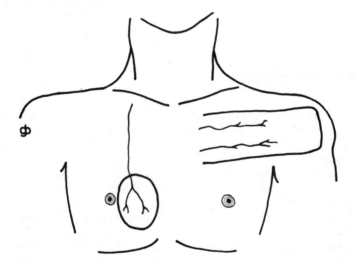

Figure 3.5 A myocutaneous flap of skin is shown on the patient's right and a delto-pectoral flap on the left with their blood supply

time these tumours are diagnosed the majority are large and require fairly extensive surgical excision. The defect that is created requires to be filled by some form of flap (*Figure 3.5*) and the patient is usually given radiotherapy in addition. Disappointingly, the cure rate from such extensive treatment is poor. Currently, chemotherapy does not increase survival but can be of value in palliation. There will remain, however, a number of patients in whom no pathology can be detected. These individuals are often concerned that they may have cancer and once it is ascertained that they do not have cancer they should be reassured. Subsequently their symptoms usually become less pressing. Symptomatic relieve can often be achieved by 'moisturizing' mouth washes, gargles or sweets containing glycerine.

Table 3.1 Commoner causes of dysphagia

Mouth	Oropharynx	Hypopharynx
No dentures	Viral pharyngitis	Viral pharyngitis
Dental caries	Tonsillitis	Anaemia
Aphthous ulcers	Carcinoma	Pharyngeal pouch
Anaemia		Muscle incoordination
Carcinoma		Neurological disease
		Carcinoma

■ Conclusions

- Difficulty in eating and the sensation of 'something being there' are symptoms of oral and pharyngeal disease.
- Actual obstruction to swallowing is more likely a symptom of oesophageal disease.
- As part of the alimentary tract mucosa, the oral mucosa often displays generalized disease, of which anaemia is the commonest.
- Clinical examination is the crux of diagnosis in the mouth and oropharynx.
- Dental problems are probably the commonest cause of difficulty in eating.
- Chronic irritation of the pharynx by cigarette smoke and dust is also common.

- Carcinoma should be rigorously sought especially in the relatively blind oral sulci.
- Asymmetry in tonsil size in an adult suggests a carcinoma and biopsy is essential.
- Hypopharyngeal disease is often diagnosed radiologically. If a hypopharyngeal tumour is a possibility, direct visualization under anaesthesia is mandatory.
- Pharyngeal pouches cause extrinsic pressure on the pharynx, are diagnosed by barium swallow and are usually surgically excised.
- Muscle incoordination of the pharynx is best diagnosed by assessment of a video recording of a barium swallow.
- Motor neuron disease of the pharynx is invariably fatal due to aspiration pneumonia. Palliation is difficult.

Nasopharynx and adenoids

Adenoid hypertrophy is the most frequent nasopharyngeal problem in children. It cannot be considered a disease as, in childhood, lymphatic tissue is normally active and appears hypertrophied when compared with the adult state. This natural hypertrophy can, however, cause symptoms by blocking off the nasal airway or by affecting Eustachian tube function. Such problems will invariably regress with time as the child's immunocompetence matures and the adenoids reduce in size. In some, however, the symptoms can be so pressing that surgical removal is indicated.

Symptoms of nasal obstruction

Many children appear to have a constantly blocked or runny nose. In most this will be due to recurrent upper respiratory tract infections and the inability of the child to blow his nose. Only in a few will adenoid hypertrophy be the cause and the difficulty is how to distinguish these from the rest. In trying to do so it is surprising how often a child, said to be a constant mouth breather, has no difficulty in breathing through his nose when his mouth is shut. In these children, mouth breathing is a habit. Inspection of the nose anteriorly should define whether there is gross mucosal oedema and mucopus but this does not clarify whether adenoid hypertrophy is a major factor. If one is fortunate, mirror examination of the postnasal space will help, but in many this is not possible due to lack of cooperation in the child. Lateral soft tissue X-rays of the postnatal space, if performed with the soft palate relaxed, can assess the bulk of the adenoids in relation to the postnasal space. However, in a specific child, it is usually a matter of clinical judgement as to the role of the adenoids in the causation of nasal obstruction.

The other nasal symptom often ascribed to adenoid hypertrophy is snoring. This is a non-fatal complaint but it does give rise to much parental concern. Snoring is most commonly caused by palatal and faucial pillar vibrations during mouth breathing rather than adenoid hypertrophy.

Symptoms of Eustachian tube dysfunction

It has been suggested that adenoid hypertrophy may cause the retention in the middle ear of mucus either by directly occluding or by preventing the opening of the Eustachian tube, creating the condition of otitis media with effusion (page 46). If this retention becomes established, the child may complain of, or be noticed to have, a hearing impairment. This will be of a conductive type because the surface tension of the mucus immobilizes the ossicular chain and the tympanic membrane.

The role of adenoid hypertrophy in otitis media with effusion is by no means proven. Otitis media with effusion certainly occurs secondarily to upper respiratory infections because of mucosal oedema of the Eustachian tube, and also when the Eustachian tube is occluded by a nasopharyngeal tumour. Otitis media with effusion is, however, exceedingly common in children with a cleft palate, in whom the condition is not created by Eustachian tube obstruction but rather by the inability of the Eustachian tube to open because of the defective palatal musculature. A defect of Eustachian tube function has naturally been postulated as a more likely cause of otitis media with effusion than adenoidal obstruction in children. Whatever the answer, there would appear to be a place for adenoidectomy in the management of otitis media with effusion.

Symptoms of palatal dysfunction

Palatal dysfunction can cause two different types of speech defect. Hyponasality occurs when the nose is unable to function as a resonant chamber when the postnasal space is full of adenoid tissue and the palate cannot relax any further to allow air into the nose. Children with hyponasal speech sound as if they have a constant cold.

Hypernasal speech occurs when the soft palate is unable to close off the postnasal space. As it is necessary to close the palate to pronounce consonants such as k, t, g, d, these sound muffled as they do in a cleft palate child. Hypernasality can occur after adenoidectomy if there is a relative shortness of the soft palate. Understandably then, adenoidectomy is contraindicated in cleft palate children and in those with a submucous cleft, which can be detected by palpating the posterior part of the hard palate.

Treatment of adenoid hypertrophy

If it is decided that the adenoid hypertrophy merits treatment because of the severity of the symptoms, the only available management is adenoidectomy under a general anaesthetic by curetting. Total removal of all adenoid tissue is impossible because of its distribution, so some patchy compensatory hypertrophy of remaining tissue is inevitable. As the indications for adenoidectomy are not the same as for tonsillectomy, there is little logic in performing adenoidectomy routinely along with tonsillectomy unless dual indications are present. Adenoidectomy is not without side effects. Postoperative haemorrhage can lead to death. In addition, the loss of adenoid bulk can cause hypernasal speech especially when there is a short palate or a submucous cleft.

■ Conclusions

- In children the adenoids are normally hypertrophied and in the majority this causes no symptoms.
- This natural adenoid hypertrophy regresses with time.
- Occasionally adenoid hypertrophy may be implicated in nasal obstruction or otitis media with effusion.
- Clinical assessment of adenoid size and extent is often difficult.
- Lateral soft tissue radiology of the postnasal space can be helpful.
- Curettage under general anaesthetic is the usual method of removal.
- Adenoidectomy can cause speech problems, due to the develop-

ment of palatal incompetence and is, therefore, contraindicated in children with a submucous or overt cleft palate.

- Adenoid hypertrophy sufficient to cause symptoms does not occur in teenagers or in adult life. In them a nasopharyngeal tumour is virtually the only diagnosis for a nasopharyngeal swelling.
- Persistent otitis media with effusion in adults suggests a nasopharyngeal tumour.

Snoring and sleep apnoea

Most adults snore occasionally, but there are those who snore habitually. Amongst this group are a few that develop obstructive sleep apnoea syndrome. This potential diagnosis has thus to be considered in all those that habitually snore.

Mechanism of snoring

Snoring is caused by a partial obstruction of the upper airway which causes vibration, most commonly of the uvula and soft palate on inspiration. An alternative site of the obstruction is at the base of the tongue and nasal obstruction may also be implicated. Snoring becomes commoner with increasing age, mainly because of increased laxity of soft tissue and the deposition of fat in the upper aero-digestive tract. Thus, overall, 25 per cent of men and 15 per cent of women are habitual snorers but the frequency doubles in those who are overweight or over 65 years of age.

Management of snoring

The main problem of snoring is a social one, many medical consultations being prompted by the patient's sleeping partner. The majority of us snore, often after excessive alcohol, so habitual drinkers are often habitual snorers. Those that are overweight should be told that their problem is due to fatty deposits in the hypopharynx. Weight loss is the way to cure this. Many also only snore whilst lying on their backs. Unfortunately, unless you are a princess, a cotton reel in the back of your pyjamas is useless but it may be worth suggesting a closely fitting tee-shirt with a pocket sewn in the back into which something as large as a tennis ball is placed.

Patients who are not obese and have a moderate alcohol intake are potential candidates for surgery if the sound originates from a vibrating uvula and soft palate. Whether this is the case can be assessed by sedating the patient to encourage snoring and then looking into the pharynx with a nasendoscope. Having confirmed the site, the uvula can be removed and the soft palate shortened by taking a strip off its edge. This is the operation of uvulopalatopharyngoplasty or U triple P (UPPP) but some caution is necessary as overenthusiastic surgery can cause nasal regurgitation of fluids and hypernasal speech.

Obstructive sleep apnoea

Every so often in snoring breathing ceases spontaneously, the individual becomes restless and moves. If these apnoeic episodes happen frequently, sleep will be sufficiently disturbed for daytime somnolence to occur. This happens at times when others would not normally fall asleep such as whilst waiting to see the doctor or driving a car. In a few, because their arterial oxygen saturation falls to below 70 per cent, pulmonary hypertension with right ventricular hypertrophy and cor-pulmonale can develop. Charles Dickens' Joe of the Pickwick Club was both obese and hypersomnolent and the description of him describes the classical full-blown syndrome.

Confirmation of the diagnosis is by overnight sleep monitoring in hospital. At its simplest the number of apnoeic episodes and the oxygen saturation levels are recorded. Sometimes, in addition, respiratory effort, nasal and oral airflow, electrocardiograms and electroencephalograms are recorded.

As with snoring, loss of weight and reduction in alcohol intake is paramount. In a few, the upper airway tract is narrowed by pathology such as a grossly deviated septum in adults or grossly hypertrophied tonsils in children. Surgery to these can give relief. If there is no obstructive pathology, management is continuous positive airway pressure during the night. This consists of wearing a tight face mask connected to a pump which ensures that the pressure in the upper airway remains positive, therefore avoiding obstruction.

■ Conclusions

• Snoring that disturbs a sleeping partner is commoner in those that are overweight and drink excessive alcohol.

- Snoring is caused most commonly by a vibrating soft palate and uvula.
- If troublesome snoring persists after weight loss and reduced alcohol intake, surgically shortening the palate can be effective.
- Obstructive sleep apnoea occurs in habitual snorers because of recurrent episodes of cessation of breathing.
- This causes daytime somnolence and sometimes right-sided heart failure.
- The initial management is as for snoring.
- Upper airway obstruction due to grossly enlarged adenoids in children and grossly deviated nasal septum in adults can contribute and should be corrected.
- Sometimes positive pressure ventilation at night or a tracheostomy is required for obstructive sleep apnoea.

The larynx

Applied anatomy

The larynx has three main functions.

1. It prevents the entry of food and saliva from the hypopharynx into the respiratory tract.
2. It produces sound vibrations which are modified by palatal, tongue and lip movements to produce speech.
3. It produces coughs.

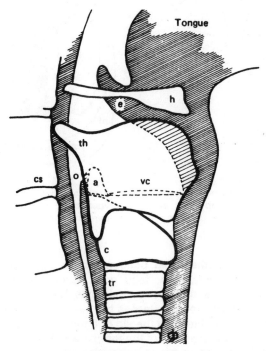

Figure 4.1 *Lateral schematic view of larynx.* a, arytenoid; c; cricoid cartilage; cs, cervical spine, e. epiglottis; vc, vocal cord; h, hyoid bone; th, thyroid cartilage; tr, tracheal cartilage; o, oesophagus

It does these by being a muscular structure within an articulating framework of the thyroid, cricoid, arytenoid and epiglottic cartilages (*Figure 4.1*). Functionally, it is divided into three parts as is illustrated in the coronal section of *Figure 4.2*.

The vocal cords, or glottis, comprise the middle part and are mainly responsible for the production of sound vibrations and coughs. The false cords, or supraglottis, are above the vocal cords and act as a sphincter to the laryngeal inlet. Their main function is to prevent food and saliva gaining access to the lower respiratory tract and this is done by a combination of its sphincteric action and laryngeal tilting. The latter occurs during swallowing due to the muscular action of the

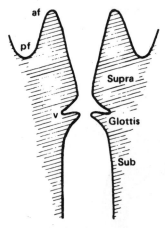

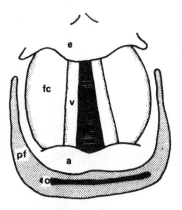

Figure 4.2 *Coronal section through the mid-larynx.* supra, supraglottis; sub, subglottis; af, aryepiglottic fold; pf, pyriform fossa; v, ventricle

Figure 4.3 *Mirror view of larynx.* a, arytenoid; e, epiglottis; fc, false vocal cord; o, oesophagus; pf, pyriform fossa; v, true vocal cord

tongue lifting up the hyoid bone which, in turn, tilts the larynx backwards. Normally, then, food goes round the larynx via the pyriform fossa rather than over the epiglottis. The subglottis is the area between the larynx and the trachea but has no specific function.

It is usually possible, with the aid of a mirror, to examine most of the larynx. Behind the base of the tongue will be seen the epiglottis (*Figure 4.3*), from which the aryepiglottic folds run posteriorly to the arytenoids, to form the laryngeal inlet. On either side are the pyriform fossae. Within the larynx it should be possible to see the false and true vocal cords with the exception of their anterior parts which can be hidden by the epiglottis.

The vagus nerve (*Figure 4.4*) is sensory to the larynx and motor to the larynx and pharynx. The sensory supply of the supraglottis is from the internal laryngeal nerve and that of the glottis and subglottis from the recurrent laryngeal nerve. The motor supply to the hypopharynx is mainly from the external laryngeal nerve and that to the supraglottis and glottis from the recurrent laryngeal nerve. Lesions of the recurrent laryngeal nerve, therefore, produce a cord palsy and loss of sensation of the vocal cord on that side. The left side is most commonly affected as that side alone enters the chest and goes below the aortic arch before returning to the larynx.

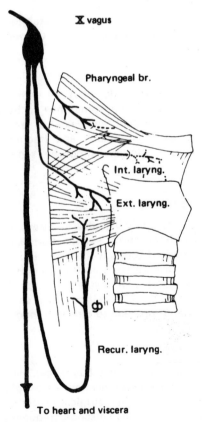

Figure 4.4 Distribution of vagus nerve to larynx

Hoarseness is primarily a symptom of glottic disease and can be caused by inflammation, neoplasia or a cord palsy. Likewise, stridor is usually a symptom of glottic disease. Neoplasia of the supra- and subglottis can cause stridor, but it is usually because it has spread to the glottis rather than that the supra- or subglottis is actually obstructed. Inhalation of food and saliva is a symptom of loss of sensation, muscle weakness or paralysis of the supraglottis which frequently is associated with similar problems of the glottis. Then the problem is, of course, much worse because of the absence of the cough reflex.

Examination of the larynx

As specialist instruments are required to examine the larynx, only those trained in their use can competently examine the larynx.

Indirect laryngoscopy

The initial examination is made indirectly with a mirror, the soft palate and oropharynx having sometimes to be sprayed with a topical anaesthetic (4 per cent lignocaine) to lessen gagging. This method of examination is difficult and frequently some areas, especially the anterior glottis, cannot be seen because of the epiglottis.

Fibreoptic laryngoscopy

This technique is particularly valuable to assess the movements of the vocal cords and if the mirror examination has been unsuccessful. The scope is passed through the nose and a topically anaesthetized palate and oropharynx into the hypopharynx from where the larynx can be viewed at rest and during phonation. Small biopsies can be taken by this method but if serious pathology is suspected it is usual to proceed to direct laryngoscopy.

Direct laryngoscopy

Under a general anaesthetic the larynx can be viewed directly, usually with microscopic magnification via a rigid scope and any suspicious areas biopsied. Microsurgical procedures such as cord stripping are performed via such a scope, frequently with the use of a CO_2 laser.

Voice disorders in adults

A voice disorder is a symptom one should never disregard as it could be the presenting symptom of a laryngeal tumour which is the commonest site for a tumour in the head and neck region. The first thing the clinician has to decide when a patient complains of problems with his voice is whether it is dysphonia or aphonia. Dysphonia is an alteration in the quality of the voice and includes hoarseness. Aphonia is a loss or weakness of the voice. Dysphonia invariably has a pathological basis whereas aphonia is most commonly psychosomatic. Having established that there is hoarseness or a change in the quality of the voice it is important to find out whether it is of recent onset or has been present for longer than two or three weeks as this dictates the management.

Acute hoarseness

Acute laryngitis is something that most individuals will have had at some time or other. It is usually due to the trauma of overusing the voice or tobacco smoke (not necessarily produced by the subject) acting on a laryngeal mucosa whose natural resistance may have been weakened by a viral upper respiratory tract infection. Hoarse voices are, therefore, common after a good party.

Acute laryngitis is usually accompanied by a slight throat discomfort which can be symptomatically relieved by saline gargles or steam inhalations. The inclusion of menthol crystals in the jug of hot water can make the latter more pleasant but no more efficacious. It should always settle down within a few days; if it does not, it is not acute laryngitis and the patient should be referred for an otolaryngological opinion.

Chronic hoarseness

It is a well founded dictum of medical practice that any adult with hoarseness, even intermittently, for longer than three weeks should be referred. This is not because the majority will have tumours but because non-otolaryngologists are unable to examine the larynx reliably with a mirror to exclude a tumour. Even otolaryngologists do not always find this easy and if they are in doubt they will almost invariably perform a fibre optic laryngoscopy or a direct examination under anaesthesia.

In taking the history the otolaryngologist will define how much the patient uses his voice, smokes or works in a dusty or otherwise traumatic atmosphere, but the diagnosis rests primarily on the clinical examination. One of the following pathologies is usually detected.

Chronic laryngitis

Chronic laryngitis is the commonest cause of chronic hoarseness. Even if a mirror examination is technically successful, it is often difficult to exclude a neoplasm as they so often arise in a localized, hyperkeratotic area in a chronically inflamed larynx. Otolaryngologists, even if they are fairly confident of a non-malignant diagnosis, will perform a direct laryngoscopy with biopsy in many of these individuals. Once a neoplasm has been excluded, chronic laryngitis is treated by avoidance of traumatizing agents, especially tobacco, and symptomatically relieved by steam inhalations.

Vocal polyps

Benign single polyps on the edge of the vocal cord are not uncommon in adults. Their endoscopic removal is under a general anaesthetic with microscopic vision is usually effective. In contrast are the more uncommon multiple polyps (*papillomatosis*) that occur in children, and present not only with hoarseness but with stridor (page 139) both of which are difficult to treat.

Vocal nodules

Vocal nodules are localized thickenings of the middle third of the vocal cord, which is the point of maximal contact during vocalization. Hence, vocal nodules are produced by overuse or maluse of the voice. The management is voice rest and instruction in the correct use of the voice by speech therapists. If this conservative management fails, the nodules can be removed utilizing microsurgical techniques.

Laryngeal tumours

Laryngeal tumours are commoner in male smokers and heavy drinkers with rotten teeth, but they can also occur in abstemious spinsters. Direct laryngoscopy under anaesthesia is necessary to assess the extent of the tumour and confirm histologically from a biopsy that it is a tumour, most often a squamous carcinoma.

If the lesion is small the cure rate with radiotherapy is high, with minimal side-effects. The larger the tumour, the less effective is radiotherapy, and some form of laryngectomy becomes the management of choice. Total laryngectomy is the most frequently performed. This necessitates a permanent tracheostomy and the loss of normal speech production. Various forms of partial laryngectomy have been tried to avoid this but others such as food aspiration are substituted. The creation of a tracheoesophageal fistula, either at the time of total laryngectomy or secondarily, has been a considerable advance regarding speech production. The

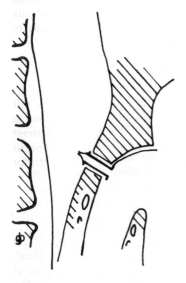

Figure 4.5 Oropharyngeal fistula with speaking valve

fistula requires a valved tube to prevent it from closing (*Figure 4.5*). On exhaling, a finger is placed over the tracheostome which diverts air via the valved tube to the oropharynx. Thus speech is possible and only varies from normal by lacking the laryngeal vibration component. Unfortunately, some cannot adjust to this method of voice production but the proportion that cannot is considerably less than those attempting the alternative of oesophageal speech. This requires the patient to learn to regurgitate swallowed air from the stomach.

Vocal cord palsy

Vocal cord palsies can be caused by lesions anywhere along the course of the vagus nerve in the neck and chest and are, therefore, commoner on the left side because of its intrathoracic course. If a cord palsy is detected the clinician's task is to try and determine the aetiology (*Table 4.1*).

Table 4.1 Aetiology of vocal cord palsy

Idiopathic	(?neuropathy)
Tumours	Chest
	Oesophagus
	Mediastinum
	Base of skull
Tuberculous scarring at lung apex	
Arteriosclerotic dilatation of aortic arch	
Surgical trauma	

The clinician's first task is to excude a neoplasm within the chest and this is done primarily by radiology and sputum cytology. Bronchoscopy and oesophagoscopy may be performed but it is unfortunately rare to be able to cure a chest tumour which is associated with a vocal cord palsy because of the size and position it will have to be before it does so. In the majority palliative therapy is all that can be done. Radiology will also detect tubercular scarring at the lung apex, the disease in most instances being healed and not requiring therapy. Arteriosclerotic dilatation of the aortic cord is again diagnosed by chest radiology. Another cause of a vocal cord palsy is damage during thyroid gland surgery but this should be obvious from the history and neck scar. Finally, a considerable proportion of individuals will have no obvious aetiology and in them if there are no other symptoms the presumptive cause is a neuropathy.

If a cause for the palsy is identified this is managed appropriately. If no cause is identified the patient is reviewed and in the majority the hoarseness will have resolved due to recovery of the palsy or to compensatory movement of the other cord. Injection of teflon paste into the cord is a simple surgical procedure which can be performed when recovery does not occur and hoarseness persists.

Dysphonia/aphonia

Intermittent weakness or loss of voice without any alteration of the quality of the voice is a psychosomatic disorder. Obviously, the larynx should be examined to exclude any coexistent pathology and if the patient has symptoms at the time of examination he or she should be asked to cough. It is surprising how often a good cough can be produced by someone with 'no voice'. The management is reassurance.

■ Conclusions

- Acute hoarseness is usually due to trauma from excess voice use and tobacco.
- Acute hoarseness should resolve within two to three weeks. If it does not it is chronic hoarseness.
- All individuals with chronic hoarseness require an otolaryngological examination with a mirror.
- Fibreoptic or direct laryngoscopy will be necessary in many to exclude a laryngeal tumour.
- Vocal nodules are managed by voice retraining and rest. Surgical removal may be necessary.
- Chronic laryngitis is managed by excluding traumatizing factors, mainly tobacco.
- Laryngeal tumours are managed by radiotherapy when small and laryngectomy when large.
- Vocal cord palsies merit investigation to exclude chest neoplasms.

Stridor

The term 'stridor' is classically used for the bovine-like inspiratory noise associated with laryngeal obstruction. This has to be differentiated from a wheeze, as in asthma, which occurs during both inspiration and expiration and is due to narrowing of the bronchioles. It also has to be differentiated from a rattle, which is due to excess secretions in the trachea. Stridor is more common in children than in adults because of the relatively small diameter of their airways, in addition to which the supporting laryngeal cartilages may be soft and collapsible (laryngomalacia) and there may be associated congenital abnormalities such as webs or haemangio-mas. In addition, they are more prone to viral infections of the mucociliary lining of the upper respiratory tract (laryngotracheo-bronchitis). If the reactive oedema is gross, obstruction at the vocal cord level may occur. Lastly, children are more likely to swallow peanuts, coins and other foreign objects which cause stridor either by direct obstruction in the larynx or by compressing the trachea when lodged in the upper oesophagus.

Adults, because of their relatively large airway, infrequently develop obstruction due to infection or foreign bodies but they are more liable to laryngeal tumours, laryngeal trauma and bilateral recurrent laryngeal nerve palsies. The first is because they smoke, the second because they are thrown against sharp edges such as a motor car dashboard and the last because they undergo thyroid surgery.

A group of patients that have to be particularly observed for stridor are those with large laryngeal tumours being treated with radiotherapy, as the reactionary oedema to this often initially increases the tumour bulk and narrows even further an already compromised airway.

Diagnosis and management

Unlike most conditions in medicine, diagnosis often has to take second place to management. In all cases clearing the airway of secretion by suction is paramount. Any dentures are removed at the same time to avoid further problems. Simple suction can often greatly relieve symptoms and although it may not eliminate the need for surgery, it can 'buy' time. Obviously if a foreign object is seen at the same time it will be removed. If severe stridor presents and if there is still an immediate danger to life one of the following must be done, the choice depending on where the emergency occurs and experience.

Laryngotomy

Stick a needle/knife between the cricoid and the thyroid cartilages and keep the hole open (*Figure 4.6*). This is most appropriate for emergencies outside a hospital and for amateur boy scouts.

Pass an endotracheal tube

This is usually the most appropriate treatment in a hospital (*Figure 4.7*), except perhaps following laryngeal trauma or when a tumour is

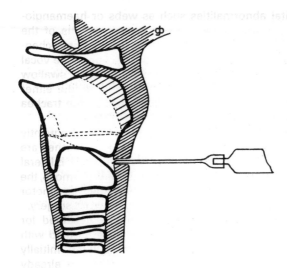

Figure 4.6 Laryngotomy

present. It is a skill all clinicians should acquire, but anaesthetists are those with the greatest experience. If the patient is *in extremis* no anaesthetic is necessary but hopefully action will be taken before then and a light inhalation anaesthetic given. Direct vision of the larynx will identify the cause of the stridor in most instances. If the cause is a foreign body it is removed. Otherwise it is usually possible to intubate the larynx past any pathology using an appropriately sized tube.

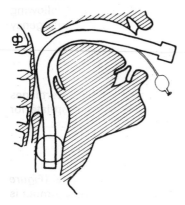

Figure 4.7 Endotracheal intubation

Perform a tracheostomy

This is easier if there already is an endotracheal tube in place, but also essential if intubation fails.

In a hospital situation both the anaesthetist and the ENT surgeon (or any surgeon that is available) should be called. If the situation is so desperate that the patient cannot wait, perform one of the above manoeuvres, remembering that it is better to have to cope with bleeding and other complications than to fill in a death certificate. If there is more time, the first specialist to arrive will probably wait for the second. Together, in a suitably equipped situation (usually an operating theatre) laryngoscopy will be performed to ascertain the pathology. Foreign bodies can be removed with immediate relief. If resolution is likely to occur within days (as in laryngotracheo-bronchitis, acute epiglottitis and overdoses) endotracheal intubation is all that is necessary. If longer-term intubation is likely, then a tracheostomy is often performed soon after intubation (*Figure 4.8*).

If laryngotomy, intubation or tracheostomy are not performed because life does not appear to be immediately at risk, it must be remembered that the clinical condition can rapidly deteriorate. In

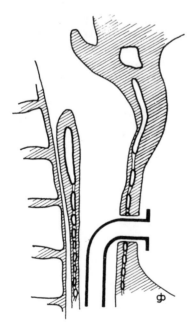

Figure 4.8 Tracheostomy

Table 4.2 Commoner causes of stridor

Infants	Laryngomalacia Congenital abnormalities
Children	Laryngotracheobronchitis (croup) Acute epiglottitis Foreign body Laryngeal papilloma
Adults	Laryngeal neoplasms Bilateral vocal cord palsy Laryngotracheobronchitis Acute epiglottitis External trauma Laryngeal/tracheal stenosis (following intubation) Foreign body

this situation it is important to have adequately trained personnel and the appropriate instruments immediately available.

Arriving at a diagnosis

Once the patient has settled it should be possible to take a history to try and identify the aetiology. *Table 4.2* is a list of the commoner causes of stridor in appropriate order of frequency for infants, children and adults as these are different in each group. It is not usually difficult to come to a diagnosis, the speed of onset and the presence of fever being particularly helpful.

Laryngomalacia

The tracheal cartilages in newborn children are particularly soft. If this is marked the negative pressure of inspiration can cause the trachea to collapse.

Congenital abnormalities

These are rare. The commonest is an anterior web between the true cords.

Laryngotracheobronchitis (croup)

The child will usually have a preceding history of an upper respiratory tract infection, often with a sore throat and hoarse voice. The majority of such infections resolve without severe symptoms developing and can, therefore, be managed at home. In some, the oedema in the subglottic region becomes so gross that the child becomes stridulous. Deaths can occur, so when suspected, hospitalization is merited. During transit to hospital, the child should be medically accompanied in case acute obstruction occurs. In children with stridor, examination of the mouth is as far as one should go. Examination of the pharynx and the larynx is contraindicated because this can precipitate obstruction. Thankfully, in hospital, the majority will settle with aspiration of secretions, humidification and nebulized adrenaline. Intubation is advised in the more severe cases and usually prednisolone is given as well.

Acute epiglottitis

This is potentially a more life-threatening condition than laryngotracheobronchitis and is due to a *Haemophilus influenzae* infection of the epiglottis. This can swell within a few hours and block off the airway causing death. Acute epiglottitis is distinguished from laryngotracheobronchitis in that it is almost invariably associated with pain and drooling of saliva. So if difficulty in breathing develops in a child and is associated with drooling or pain, emergency action is required and, in particular, early intubation. Thereafter the management is along the lines suggested for laryngotracheobronchitis but includes intravenous antibiotics, most commonly chloramphenicol or a third generation cephalosporin, e.g. cefotaxime.

Though epiglottitis is less common in adults, difficulty in breathing associated with pain and difficulty in swallowing still merits emergency action because death can occur.

Foreign bodies

Here the child is well one minute and stridulous the next. Often this will occur while they are eating but equally what they have inhaled may not be obvious. If the child is small enough to be held upside down by the feet, it is given a slap on the back. Otherwise a quick bear hug around the abdomen (Heimlich manoeuvre) will raise the diaphragm causing a sudden exhalation, hopefully with the foreign body. If this is not successful endoscopic removal is necessary.

Laryngeal papillomatosis

This is primarily a childhood condition which can be difficult to treat. The papillomas are akin to warts on the larynx and recurrence is common. Surgical removal by avulsion, or perhaps better by CO_2

laser excision, has often to be repeated. Topical preparations such as podophyllin can have a role. Natural resolution will occur over years but until this occurs, some may require a speaking tracheostomy (page 146).

Laryngeal trauma

Mainly because of legislation requiring the wearing of seat belts, laryngeal trauma from being thrown against a car dashboard with the neck extended is now relatively rare.

Laryngeal neoplasia

See page 136. A CO_2 laser can be used temporarily to debulk a large tumour to alleviate stridor.

■ Conclusions

- Stridor is life threatening and management often takes precedence over diagnosis.
- The airway should first be cleared of secretions and false teeth.
- Any obstructing foreign body is removed as soon as it is identified.
- Laryngotomy, tracheostomy or endotracheal intubation should be performed sooner rather than later.
- Children are particularly at risk because of the relatively small size of their airways.
- In them acute epiglottitis and laryngotracheobronchitis can be life threatening.
- The presence of drooling and/or pain usually distinguishes acute epiglottitis from laryngotracheobronchitis.
- In adults acute epiglottitis can also be fatal.
- In the non-emergency situation, humidification and continued aspiration of secretions is beneficial.
- Antibiotics, usually ampicillin, are indicated for acute epiglottitis and laryngotracheobronchitis.
- Inhaled foreign bodies in the larynx cause acute stridor. A slap on the back will hopefully expel it if the child can be held upside down by the legs.
- A bear hug around the abdomen is the emergency treatment for inhaled foreign bodies in those too big to be suspended by their legs.

Tracheostomy

There are three main indications for a tracheostomy each having a different likely duration. Firstly, it may be required short term to relieve acute airway obstruction until this settles down usually within days (page 140). Secondly, it may be required medium term in the management of lung failure for up to a couple of weeks to bypass the dead space of the upper respiratory tract. Thirdly, it may be required long term when a narrowed laryngeal inlet is unlikely to resolve such as with a stricture or following partial laryngectomy.

In these three types of situation, a tracheostomy tube is primarily required to keep the stoma open otherwise it will almost invariably close. This does not occur when the larynx has been totally excised. Hence a tube is usually unnecessary in patients with a total laryngectomy.

Over the years many different designs and different materials have been used in the manufacture of tracheostomy tubes. At present plastic and silastic are the materials most commonly used. In general the features selected are those appropriate to the likely duration of intubation (*Table 4.3*).

Table 4.3 Tracheostomy tube design features

	Duration intubation		
	Short term	*Medium term*	*Long term*
Tube features	Single Plastic ? Cuffed	Single Plastic Cuffed	Double Silastic Valved
Object of intubation	Acute airway obstruction	Lung failure	Permanently narrowed or absent larynx

Design features of tracheostomy tubes
(*Figure 4.9* and *Table 4.3*)

General features

An introducer aids the insertion of all types of tracheostomy tube but obviously has to be removed immediately the tube is in place to allow breathing.

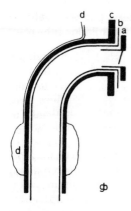

Figure 4.9 *Design features that are available in various combinations on tracheostomy tubes.* a, speaking valve; b, inner tube; c, outer tube; d, inflatable cuff

Short term tubes

A single non-cuffed plastic tube is all that is required, though some might use a cuffed tube to prevent blood trickling down the trachea postoperatively. It is better to secure haemostasis.

Medium term tubes

Initially in lung failure, it is usual to deliver positive pressure ventilation via a cuffed endotracheal tube. In the conscious patient, after a few days, it is more comfortable to change to a cuffed tracheostomy tube if ventilation is to be continued for more than a few days. The object of the cuff is to prevent the escape of air/gases back out of the trachea during the positive phase of ventilation. The cuff is *not* used to prevent the tube falling out – tapes do that. The cuff should only be inflated to the point where it just occludes the tracheal lumen. Inflation to a point greater than this may cause pressure necrosis of the mucosa and perhaps the tracheal cartilage, which almost invariably leads to tracheal stenosis. Fortunately, recent advances in cuff design have made this less of a problem than formerly. The two main alternatives are foam or high volume and low pressure cuffs which are not deflated once the correct degree of inflation is achieved.

How then is the correct degree of cuff inflation achieved? It is not by injecting a certain volume of air, as each individual trachea has a different diameter. It is not by assessing the pressure in the indicator balloon, as the pressure in this does not reflect the pressure within the cuff because of differing elasticity. The correct method is to inflate the cuff until there is no escape of air or gases detected past the cuff and then slowly to deflate it until escape is just detected. The cuff is then at the right pressure, and, unless a one way valve is being used, artery forceps are then applied to the inflation tube prior to removing the syringe and inserting the bung.

Long term tubes

Non-cuffed tubes are preferred in circumstances other than with positive pressure ventilation. If there is no cuff, there is no danger of cuff complications. Double tubes have a distinct advantage in long term usage regarding cleaning. The inner tube is marginally longer than the outer tube and, therefore, any crusting of secretions occurs on the inner tube. This can then be removed for cleaning, the outer tube remaining in position in the tracheostome. Single tubes have to be removed in their entirety for cleaning and have to be reinserted, which apart from being tedious, can traumatize the trachea. Valved tubes are used where the larynx is still *in situ* to allow the patient to speak. Valves are used less frequently than they might be and thereby unnecessary psychological and communication problems are created. The valve is a hinged trapdoor that is inserted at the opening of the inner tube so that inspired air gains easy access. On expiration the valve shuts and the air exits via the larynx, making speech possible. Naturally, a valved tube will not function where there is gross laryngeal obstruction or the larynx has been removed, but the degree of obstruction that will allow relatively easy expiration is often surprising. It is, of course, inspiration rather than expiration that is the main problem in laryngeal obstruction and the tracheostomy overcomes this problem.

Tracheostomy care

In an individual with a tracheostomy the inspired air is no longer humidified and warmed by the upper respiratory passages. The bronchial secretions thereby become excessively thick and sticky and respiratory complications are common unless guarded against.

In the initial stages humidification is vital and is achieved by placing a mask over the tracheostome and moist air is delivered from a nebulizer or water trap. If the tracheostomy is going to be permanent this method of humidification can gradually be discontinued and a laryngectomy bib substituted. This is a foam filled bib which is worn round the neck over the stoma and compensates to some extent for the nose. With the passage of time, even this may become unnecessary particularly as it can interfere with tracheo-oesophageal speech (page 137).

The other problem is that the patient is unable to cough up thick mucus secretions so in the initial stages regular aspiration of the secretions with a suction catheter has to be performed. Physiotherapy is also important to clear the more peripheral alveoli of secretions. Secretions often build up in the tube and this is where the double tube has its advantages, since it can be cleaned without taking the tube out completely. Single tubes have to be regularly removed for cleaning and, apart from being more time consuming, it is also uncomfortable for the patient.

■ Conclusions

- A tracheostomy can be for short, medium or long term use.
- The type of tube selected is mainly dependent on the above.
- Short term use is usually to relieve acute airway obstruction and a single plastic tube, perhaps with a cuff, is used.
- Medium term use is usually with positive pressure ventilation to assist lung function. For this, a cuffed tube is essential to allow the lungs to be inflated.
- The main danger of a cuff is tracheal stenosis. The correct cuff pressure is thus important.
- Long term use is where the laryngeal inlet is severely compromised and this is likely to persist. A non-cuffed double silastic tube eases cleaning as only the inner tube requires to be removed. A speaking valve can also be used.
- In all tracheostomy care is important. Crusting can be lessened by humidification.
- A tracheostomy lessens the ability to cough up secretions. Humidification keeps these loose. Suction aspiration is often required.
- Patients with a permanent tracheostomy, following total laryngectomy, seldom require a tube to keep the stoma open.
- In other circumstances, spontaneous closure is inevitable if a tube is not used.

How to perform a temporary tracheostomy

1. Preferably first pass an endotracheal tube.
2. Hyperextend neck by placing something beneath the shoulders.
3. Horizontal or vertical skin and subcutaneous tissue incision centred two fingerbreadths below thyroid cartilage and two fingerbreadths above sternal notch.
4. By blunt dissection open a vertical plane in the midline between the strap muscles.
5. Retract strap muscles.
6. If thyroid isthmus is in the way, either retract it or divide between two clamping forceps.

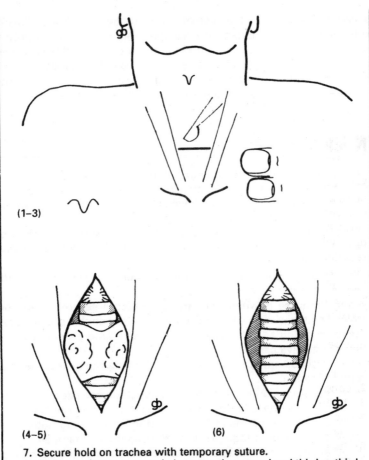

(1–3)

(4–5)

(6)

7. Secure hold on trachea with temporary suture.
8. Divide trachea transversely between the second and third *or* third and fourth tracheal cartilages. Alternatively a vertical incision can be made.

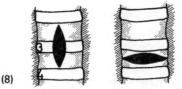

(8)

9. Aspirate blood and mucus from trachea.
10. Insert appropriately sized tracheostomy tube.
11. Tie retaining tracheostomy tapes with the neck flexed.

Figure 4.10 How to perform a temporary tracheostomy

Head and neck

Neck lumps

When a patient presents saying he has a lump or swelling in his neck, a long list of potential causes has to be considered to help find out what it is. In the majority of individuals there are always several clues from the history and from the examination of the head and neck which will allow the correct diagnosis to be made without resorting to the attitude that the easiest way to find out what the lump is is to take it out. This attitude is incorrect and, if practised haphazardly, can lead to iatrogenic spread of tumours.

The first thing that the clinician wants to know is where the swelling is. This will tell him the most likely organ or structure involved and thereafter he has to decide what the pathology is in that particular organ or structure. Essentially the lump can be in:

1. the skin and subcutaneous tissues
2. congenital remnants
3. the thyroid gland
4. the salivary glands
5. the bony and cartilaginous structures (larynx, trachea, spine)
6. the blood vessels or
7. the lymph nodes.

If it were not for the fact that there are lymph nodes everywhere in the neck, a decision as to what organ or structure is involved would be easier.

Skin

Swellings in the skin and subcutaneous structures such as sebaceous cysts and lipomas should be readily identified by the ability to lift up the mass in the skin. If necessary, these lesions are excised in total and will concern us no further.

Congenital remnants

Thyroglossal and branchial cleft cysts are the two commonest congenital cysts but even these are relatively uncommon. Surprisingly for congenital lesions, they do not usually present until the patient is in the teens or twenties, probably because it is only when they become secondarily infected or when there is haemorrhage into them that they present. Both cysts have classic positions.

Thyroglossal cysts can be anywhere along the line of development of the thyroid between the base of the tongue and the thyroid itself. Occasionally there is an associated fistula, due to the cyst having burst. Treatment is surgical excision of the cyst and its tract.

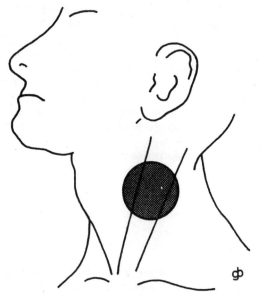

Figure 5.1 Classic situation for a branchial cyst

Branchial cysts, considered an abnormality of fusion of the branchial clefts, are classically situated in the region of the middle third of the sternomastoid muscle (*Figure 5.1*). This also is a fairly common site for an enlarged mid-cervical lymph gland. There is obviously a differential diagnosis to be made and the factors which have to be considered are discussed below.

Thyroid gland

The normal gland is impalpable here; any identifiable thyroid swelling must be considered pathological.

Swellings of the thyroid gland have a classic position around the trachea, below the thyroid cartilage (*Figure 5.2*). The thyroid is normally attached to the pretracheal fascia and when the trachea and larynx are lifted up by muscle action of the tongue on the hyoid bone during swallowing, thyroid lumps also move up. This can make them easier to palpate. The relatively rare alternative causes of a swelling in the region of the thyroid gland are pre- and paratracheal lymph nodes, which will also move on swallowing.

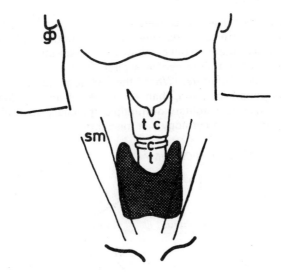

Figure 5.2 *Position of the thyroid gland.* c, cricoid; t, trachea; tc, thyroid cartilage; sm, sternomastoid muscle

Thyroid swellings can affect the whole gland or present as a single or multiple nodule. In addition, the patient may be euthyroid, thyrotoxic or hypothyroid (myxoedema). The differentiation between the various thyroid activity states can be made clinically, biochemically or by radioactive iodine uptake. Several clinical combinations can thus result but the initial differentiation is made on what type of swelling is detected.

Whole gland enlargement

Physiological enlargement in adolescents is not uncommon. This is usually visible rather than palpable.

Multinodular goitres are associated with normal thyroid function, the whole gland having a nodular feel though one lobe is often more affected. Surgical excision gives symptomatic relief if the goitre is causing pressure symptoms on the respiratory or alimentary tracts.

Hashimoto's disease The gland is diffusely enlarged secondary to autoimmune thyroiditis which is diagnosed serologically. Thyroxine or surgical excision is the management.

Solitary nodules

The majority of these are caused by benign cysts or adenomas. Some, however, are tumours. Fine needle aspiration will diagnose cysts. This will be curative but cytology on the aspirate must be done to exclude a tumour. Fine needle aspiration of a solid nodule will identify definite tumours. When the cytology is indefinite or suggests a simple oedema, than an isotope scan will determine whether the nodule is solitary or multiple. If solitary open biopsy is suggested as aspirate cytology can miss tumours.

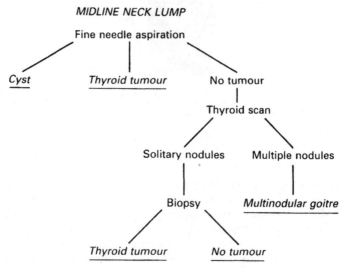

Flow Chart 8 Midline neck lump

Salivary glands

There are two, main paired salivary glands, the parotid and submandibular, that require consideration. Both have classic positions but, once again, there are lymph nodes in the same position which can cause confusion.

The parotid gland is much more extensive than commonly realized (*Figure 5.7*). The part of the gland that is often forgotten about is below the angle of the jaw, and this can be confused with swellings in the upper cervical (jugulo-digastric) lymph nodes (*Figure 5.5*). Swellings in the remainder of the parotid cause little diagnostic difficulty as to the organ they are in.

The cause of a parotid swelling is relatively easy to decide – inflammatory pathologies cause a painful tender swelling, and, with rare exceptions, all the others are neoplasms (see page 162).

The submandibular gland again has a classic situation, below the middle of the jaw (*Figure 5.3*). Swellings in this region should always be bimanually palpated, with one hand in the submandibular region and a finger of the other hand in the alveolar-lingual sulcus. This

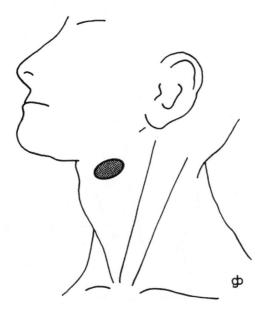

Figure 5.3 Classic position for the submandibular gland

allows the mass to be better felt and also allows stones within the duct to be identified.

Obstruction of submandibular gland secretions either by stones or 'grit' is its commonest pathology, and a history of an intermittent, painful swelling below the jaw made worse on eating or thinking of eating is classic. Radiology, either straight or with contrast dye injected into the duct, is usually helpful. The treatment is either excision of the stone when it is palpable in the duct or total removal of the submandibular gland. In this area the alternative diagnosis is a submandibular lymph gland (*Figure 5.5*). These are relatively rare, except when there is an oral tumour with secondary spread or dental caries with inflammatory lymph gland reaction. A good oral examination is, therefore, mandatory in all patients with a sub-mandibular swelling.

Bone and cartilage

The inexperienced clinician often mistakes the normal bony or cartilaginous structures in the neck for pathological lumps. The most common structure to be confused, especially in thin necks, is the

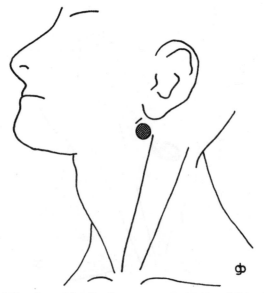

Figure 5.4 Classic position for the transverse process of the axis

transverse process of the axis which is deep below the angle of the jaw (*Figure 5.4*). The transverse processes are, of course, bilateral but one can be more prominent than the other. Other normal structures such as the hyoid bone, the thyroid and cricoid cartilages should not be difficult to identify. An accessory cervical rib can sometimes be palpable.

Blood vessels

Normally the carotid artery is not palpable, although pulsations within it are. Arteriosclerotic thickening of the wall often makes the artery palpable and the pulsations within it less so. A bruit can often be heard by auscultation over an arteriosclerotically narrowed carotid artery, although transmitted bruits from the proximal larger vessels have to be excluded by listening to them as well. Carotid body tumours are extremely rare and do not usually enter into the differential diagnosis of a lump in the neck. They classically present in the region of the carotid bifurcation.

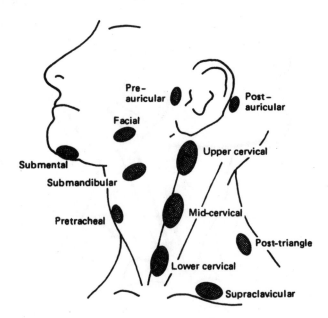

Figure 5.5 Classic pattern of distribution of neck lymph nodes

Lymph nodes

There are several hundred lymph nodes on each side of the neck. In adults, lymph nodes are not normally palpable and should be investigated. In children and adolescents it is normal to be able to palpate some lymph glands, mainly because they are chronically inflamed due to the repeated upper respiratory and alimentary tract infections in this age group. Lymph node enlargement in them need not usually arouse too much concern.

The lymph nodes, although generously distributed have a definite pattern of distribution (*Figure 5.5*), the only groups which are inaccessible to palpation being the retropharyngeal nodes. Their pattern of drainage from the different areas of the head and neck is also relatively constant (*Figure 5.6*), although in any disease process not all nodes in the chain draining the affected part are necessarily affected. Thus, an inflammatory lesion at the tip of the tongue may involve only a lower cervical lymph node.

If a lymph node is enlarged it implies pathology in the head and neck region, the only exception being the supraclavicular nodes.

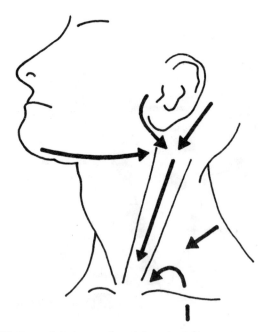

Figure 5.6 Pattern of drainage of neck lymph nodes

These nodes also drain from the thorax and, in addition, on the left there is drainage from the upper abdomen because of the relationship to the thoracic duct. The function of the lymph nodes, as anywhere in the body, is to provide a local defence mechanism against inflammation of any type, most commonly infective or neoplastic. The clinician's task is usually to differentiate between these and to define the primary site of the infection or neoplasm.

Lymph node enlargement due to infection

Lymph node enlargements which are secondary to inflammation are, or at some time have been, painful. Often several glands are affected and they usually are, or at some stage have been, tender to palpation. The most common sites to be infected are the teeth, nose and pharynx. Correspondingly, the upper cervical (jugulodigastric) lymph glands are the ones most commonly affected. As stated earlier, palpable lymph nodes are common in children, who normally have recurrent upper respiratory and oropharyngeal infections.

In adolescents, infectious mononucleosis must be considered. Here the lymphadenopathy is usually multiple and bilateral and can involve lymph gland groups apart from those of the head and neck.

In adults infective enlargement of a lymph node is uncommon and neoplasm is the more likely possibility. Primary tuberculosis of the neck nodes is however still a possibility following ingestion of the organisms and is not necessarily associated with pulmonary tuberculosis. Recent immigrants from the developing nations are particularly at risk and, as the infection is chronic, the nodes are not usually tender. Occasionally, cervical tuberculosis may present as an abscess or as a fistula, but more often the diagnosis is arrived at histologically when the node is excised to exclude a neoplasm.

Lymph node enlargement due to neoplasm

In adults, an enlarged lymph node in the neck must be considered a neoplasm until proven otherwise. In adults under the age of 40, the most likely neoplasm is a lymphoma. In those over 40, it is likely to be a secondary from a primary squamous carcinoma from somewhere in the head and neck.

In all patients the first thing to do is to examine thoroughly the head and neck, paying particular attention to other lymphatic tissue in the tonsils, the postnasal space and the base of the tongue. The area which primarily drains to the enlarged node should be examined but not to the exclusion of the other areas. The primary site for a squamous carcinoma is very often silent, that is without symptoms or signs. This is not surprising as the head and neck have many spaces where a neoplasm has to be fairly big before it causes symptoms. Examples of such spaces are the nasopharynx, the pyriform fossae, the supraglottis, the base of tongue, the tonsil and the oral cavity. The majority of these sites are not easy to examine and it should, therefore, be the rule that an otolaryngologist should examine every adult with a neck swelling. Having completed the examination, the otolaryngologist will be faced with one of two situations which are handled in different ways.

1. *Obvious primary with secondary lymph node involvement* Endoscopy to assess the extent of the primary tumour and biopsy of it to confirm the diagnosis will be carried out. The neck node can usually be assumed to be a secondary but if in doubt a fine needle aspiration may be performed. An open biopsy is not performed as this has the risk of disseminating the tumour to the skin. A pathological diagnosis of squamous carcinoma having been achieved, the primary and secondary tumours are surgically removed *en bloc*, as this gives the best chance of cure.
2. *Node(s) with no obvious primary* If reliable cytology is available, fine needle aspiration should separate out secondary tumours from lymphomas and non-specific chronic inflammation. If a secondary endoscopy under a general anaesthetic of the entire upper alimentary and respiratory tract will be carried out in

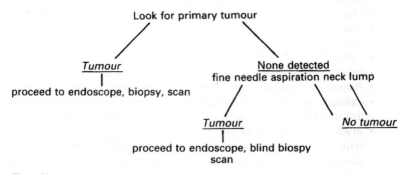

LATERAL NECK LUMP

Look for primary tumour

Tumour
|
proceed to endoscope, biopsy, scan

None detected
fine needle aspiration neck lump

Tumour
|
proceed to endoscope, blind biospy
scan

No tumour

Flow Chart 9 Lateral neck lump

search of a small primary such as in the postnasal space. If a squamous carcinoma is identified block neck dissection, to cure the obvious tumour, and radiotherapy to the head and neck, to treat what is assumed to be an occult primary, is given. If a lymphoma is identified, the liver, spleen, abdominal lymph nodes and the marrow are assessed to stage the tumour. Radiotherapy is usually given to disease localized in the head and neck and chemotherapy given for generalized disease. If only non-specific reactive changes are histologically present and there is no obvious source for the inflammation, for example in the teeth, nothing further is done.

The otolaryngologist himself will normally not be happy to exclude a primary neoplasm without performing a direct examination of all these areas under a general anaesthetic.

It is generally considered better to biopsy the primary site rather than the secondarily involved lymph node as this can lead to further local spread. When there are multiple lymph node enlargements, either on one or both sides of the neck, the neoplasm is often one of the reticuloses, for example Hodgkin's disease.

■ Conclusions

- Neck masses can be in the skin, congenital remnants, the thyroid or salivary glands, the bony or cartilaginous structures or the lymph nodes.
- The site of the mass will usually distinguish the tissue of origin.
- The age of the patient, the history and a full ENT examination will usually distinguish between the various pathologies.
- Lymph nodes are the commonest neck masses.
- Inflammatory nodes usually are or have been tender.
- Palpable lymph nodes in children are normal.
- Palpable lymph nodes in adults, unless residual from childhood, are definitely pathological.
- In an adult over 40 years of age, the cause of enlargement of a neck lymph node is most commonly neoplasm in the head and neck. A competent and thorough ENT examination is, therefore, required.

Parotid swellings

Normally the parotid is inpalpable here and any swelling must be considered pathological. Swellings in the area of the parotid gland (*Figure 5.7(a)*) are often not as easy to diagnose and identify as one might hope. Parotid swellings are often only intermittently present and they can be confused with lymph glands, both in front of the ear and over the facial vessels (*Figure 5.5*, page 157). It must also be remembered that the tail of the parotid extends below the angle of the jaw so that parotid pathology can present as a 'lump' in the neck. The parotid also extends medial to the masseter and buccinator muscles and can present as an intra-oral swelling in the region of the tonsils (*Figure 5.7(b)*). To reach a diagnosis the usual clinical history

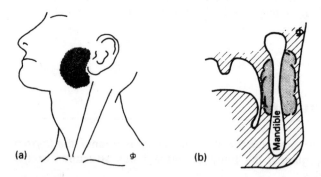

Figure 5.7 (a) Normal anatomical position of the parotid gland. (b) Location of the parotid around mandible

and examination will be performed. These can be of help, but in coming to a pathological diagnosis the main consideration will be whether the swelling is acute, intermittent or chronic. In addition, whether the swelling is painful or tender to touch and whether the swelling is unilateral or bilateral is helpful (*Table 5.1*). Tumours are more likely also if only part of the gland is involved.

Table 5.1

Parotid swellings	Pain/tenderness	Bilateral
Acute		
Mumps	x	x
Bacterial parotitis	x	–
Intermittent		
Stones	x	–
Autoimmune disease	x	x
Chronic		
Tumours	–	–

Acute swellings

These are the easiest to diagnose and are usually due to either viral or bacterial infections causing an acute parotitis.

Mumps is the commonest virus aetiology, easily identified by bilateral occurrence of painful, diffusely enlarged glands and perhaps by the dreaded complication of orchitis, pancreatitis or deafness. Mumps is treated expectantly and hopefully prevented by immunization.

Bacterial parotitis is rare, but should be thought of in ill, dehydrated patients that develop an acutely painful unilateral parotid swelling.

Persistent swellings

A persistent unilateral parotid swelling is almost certainly a tumour, particularly if only part of the gland is involved. Most frequently the tumours are benign, pleomorphic, adenomas. Unfortunately, unless there is a facial palsy, skin ulceration or grossly enlarged cervical lymph nodes, it is difficult to determine clinically which parotid tumours are malignant. The majority of both benign and malignant tumours are pain free. In the majority the initial management is superficial parotidectomy rather than biopsy or enucleation and this will cure a benign tumour. If malignancy is then detected histologically, total parotidectomy with sacrifice of the facial nerve is usually performed as radiotherapy has little part to play in most parotid tumours.

Intermittent swellings

By this is meant periodic enlargement of the parotid gland which may or may not reduce to a normal size in between.

Autoimmune disease

These cause intermittent, bilateral parotid enlargement, most often in middle-aged women. There can be manifestations of other autoimmune diseases and certain combinations have been given syndrome titles. The commonest is Sjögren's syndrome, which is a triad of intermittent parotid swelling associated with dry eyes (keratoconjunctivitis) and rheumatoid arthritis. The volume of lacrimation is reduced when measured by Schirmer's test, in which the tears are absorbed by a strip of filter or litmus paper hooked into the inferior fornix of the eye. The condition is usually progressive with the decreased salivary secretion producing a dry mouth (xerostomia) and gross dental caries in the dentulous patient. As in some autoimmune disorders, progression to lymphoma can occur. The diagnosis is confirmed by serology.

If neoplasia can be excluded treatment is expectant, steroids having a minimal part to play. If there is doubt about the diagnosis or if symptoms are severe, parotidectomy can be performed.

Stones

Parotid stones are uncommon compared with ones in the sub-mandibular salivary glands, but are suggested when the swelling is associated with preprandial discomfort. The stone can usually be palpated unless it is embedded in the gland, from which it may be milked by manual palpation. More commonly small particles of 'grit' can cause intermittent parotid swelling but, because they are impalpable, they are diagnosed by sialography. Radio-opaque dye is injected through a cannula into the parotid duct which outlines the ducts and readily identifies any obstruction. If there has been an associated intermittent low grade infection there may be fibrotic narrowing of the ducts with distal dilatation; *sialectasis*. The treatment of stones is surgical removal. Swellings due to grit particles usually improve following radiology because this has washed them out.

■ Conclusions

- Bilateral acute parotid swellings are most commonly due to mumps.
- A unilateral, acute parotid swelling is most likely due to acute parotitis.
- Persistent parotid swellings are tumours. They are usually painless and, because the majority are benign, superficial parotidectomy is diagnostic and curative for most of them.
- Intermittent parotid swellings can be due to either autoimmune disease, duct stones or grit.

Pain in the head and neck

Facial pain is a symptom that clinicians often find more difficult to diagnose than should be the case. A large proportion of individuals with facial pain do not have any identifiable pathology and the clinician often feels he has to ascribe an unjustifiable title such as sinusitis or eye strain. This can cause considerable confusion and mismanagement but the problem can be logically managed by taking a good history and by thoroughly examining the ear, nose and mouth. The causal pathology, if any, will then in most instances be identified without recourse to investigations.

Pain in the head and neck can originate in any of the head and neck structures, but these are all supplied by one of two nerves. The V cranial nerve (*Figure 5.8*) is sensory to the skin of the face, neck and ear, to the mucosa of the nose, sinuses and oral cavity and anterior two-thirds of the tongue and to the teeth. The IX cranial nerve (*Figure 5.9*) is sensory to the pharynx (naso, oro- and hypopharynx), posterior one-third of the tongue, Eustachian tube and middle ear. Pain can be either localized to the site of the disease or can be referred. When trying to identify the pathology one must, therefore, look first where the patient complains of the pain. If there is local disease there will usually be signs of inflammation and tenderness to touch. If no pathology is detected, then the clinician must examine elsewhere to exclude the causes of referred pain. Thus, if pain is complained of in the ear, the ear is first examined and if no local pathology is detected the areas of distribution of both the V and IV cranial nerves, from which the ear receives a sensory

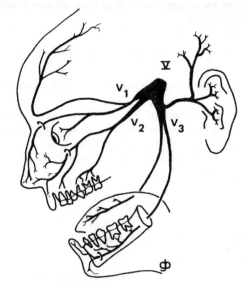

Figure 5.8 Sensory distribution of the three branches (V_1, V_2, V_3) of the V (trigeminal) cranial nerve

supply have to be examined. Referred pain is probably as common, if not commoner, than locally produced pain.

The following is a discussion of head and neck diseases which can cause pain and they will be considered primarily as causing local

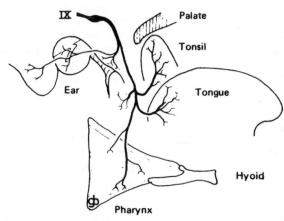

Figure 5.9 Sensory distribution of IX (glossopharyngeal) cranial nerve

pain but it must be remembered that they all can present as pain elsewhere in the head and neck.

Inevitably some of the commonest sites of pain have merited separate sections. Otalgia is covered on page 34, painful oral lesions on page 110, and sore throats on page 113.

Frontal headache

Frontal headaches are extremely common but sinusitis is an uncommon cause. In the majority no definable cause can be identified. Chronic sinusitis is invariably associated with nasal discharge: a patient without a clear cut relationship between frontal headaches and nasal discharge is unlikely to be suffering from sinusitis. Very rarely the frontal sinus ostum will become blocked and acute *frontal sinusitis* develops. This condition is usually dramatic in onset and there will be acute tenderness over the frontal bone. Antibiotics and drainage are the mainstay of management.

Temporal arteritis is another rare cause of frontal headaches. Here a tender thickened arterial wall in the temple region may be palpated. The pain is thus unilateral and the diagnosis confirmed by a high ESR which is indicative of an autoimmune condition.

Pain between the eyes and over the cheeks

In the majority of individuals with pain between the eyes and over the cheeks neither a local nor a referred cause can be identified. Idiopathic pain is, therefore, the commonest diagnosis but should only be ascribed once the recognized causes have been excluded.

The ethmoid and maxillary sinuses, when affected by acute sinusitis, cause severe local discomfort, readily identified by tenderness on local pressure and perhaps secondary soft tissue oedema of the overlying tissues. Mucopus will usually be evident in the nose. Chronic sinusitis can cause pain in these areas but it is extremely rare to have chronic sinusitis without mucopurulent rhinorrhoea and without clinical evidence of infection in the nose.

Ophthalmological causes of facial pain are uncommon, although eye tests are often recommended. Uncorrected errors of refraction can cause discomfort but should only be diagnosed if it is brought about by prolonged use of the eyes in otherwise poor visual circumstances such as poor lighting.

Trigeminal neuralgia is usually diagnosed by its episodic occurrence, its severity, its area of distribution of the trigeminal nerve, the presence of triggering factors such as eating and by its dramatic response to carbamazepine (Tegretol).

Pains in the nose

Boils of the skin in the vestibule of the nose cause acute pain but are readily identifiable.

Some individuals complain of a sensation of burning or discomfort in the nose, A local traumatic factor such as spectacles should be considered but in many cases no reason will be identified.

Occipital headache

Cervical osteoarthritis is extremely common and can cause pain either on movement of the neck or because of the secondary muscular spasm. Clinical examination of the neck should detect osteoarthritis by the lack of movement and also by triggering of the discomfort which, on occasions, may radiate down the arm. Radiology is of minimal value as the majority of normal adults will have some evidence of cervical osteoarthritis, whether or not this is causing symptoms.

Pain in the neck

Inflamed cervical lymph glands are the commonest cause of pain, and the glands will be palpable and tender. Occasionally a neck abscess can develop from a lymph gland. These will all be secondary to infection elsewhere in the head and neck and the site of origin should be carefully looked for.

Pharyngitis and laryngitis, most often viral in origin, may be felt mainly as a discomfort in the neck rather than the throat. Here there will be tenderness on palpation of the pharynx or larynx which is made worse on movement of these structures.

■ Conclusions

- Facial pain is often idiopathic, but local and referred causes of pain must be excluded.
- Otalgia is more often referred rather than locally derived pain.
- Sinusitis without nasal symptoms or signs is an extremely rare cause of facial pain.
- Facial pain is rarely caused by eyestrain, unless the history clearly suggests that it is only associated with the use of the eyes.

Bashed face

Traditionally faciomaxillary injuries are classified as to whether they primarily affect the upper (skull), middle (facial) or lower (mandibular) thirds of the head (*Figure 5.10*). Within each third, various bones or combination of bones, may be fractured. The two

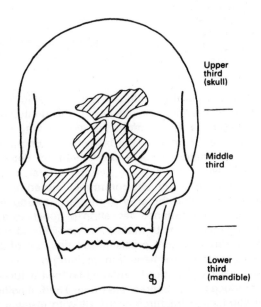

Upper
third
(skull)

Middle
third

Lower
third
(mandible)

Figure 5.10 Classification of sites of faciomaxillary injuries

commonest fractures are nasal and skull and these are dealt with elsewhere (pages 89 and 174). Thankfully, gross middle third of face fractures are now less common because the wearing of safety belts prevents the head hitting the dashboard or windscreen. Sports injuries (from a ball, racket, stick, opponent's head or fist) are more common but thankfully usually less serious.

In general, clinical observation can be extremely useful in determining whether there actually is a fracture, as opposed to soft tissue bruising. When palpating to elicit local tenderness over a potential fracture site, knowledge of the usual sites of fracture is

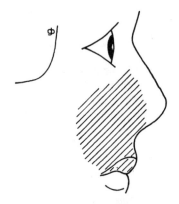

Figure 5.11 Sensory area supplied by infra-orbital nerve

extremely useful. Intra-oral examination is also most important. The interrelationship of the teeth or the jaw in the dentulous patient should be assessed as this is often the easiest way to detect a displaced mandible or middle third fractures. Enquiries about diplopia and examination of eye movement to detect muscle entrapment will usually detect any serious orbital involvement. Finally, as the infra-orbital nerve is commonly injured by a fracture, it is important to examine the area of the face it supplies (*Figure 5.11*) and compare the patient's sensation of touch to a piece of cotton wool over this area with that on the non-injured side.

Radiology determines more precisely the position of a fracture and hence is of considerable benefit in deciding the management. Repeat radiological examination to ensure that the fracture has been satisfactorily reduced is, of course, essential. The following are the signs of the commoner fractures not dealt with elsewhere, along with an indication of how they are most frequently managed.

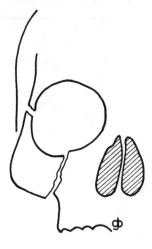

Figure 5.12 Zygomatic fractures

Zygomatic fracture (*Figure 5.12*)

Signs

1. Orbital margin step.
2. Flattened cheek, especially when viewed from above.
3. Possible asymmetry of eyes with resultant diplopia.
4. Possible infra-orbital nerve paraesthesia.

Management

Manipulative reduction via an incision at the hairline in front of the ear. After reduction, if it is unstable, wiring or plating is used.

Blow out orbital fracture (*Figure 5.13*)

Signs

Limited eye movement due to trapping of orbital muscles by the fragmented bone.

Management

Open reduction via the orbit or maxillary antrum.

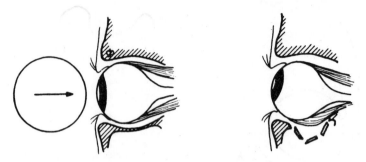

Figure 5.13 Blow out fracture of orbital floor

Le Fort fractures (*Figure 5.14*)

Signs

1. Flattened face often with potentially fatal airway obstruction.
2. Non-alignment of upper and lower dentition or jaws.

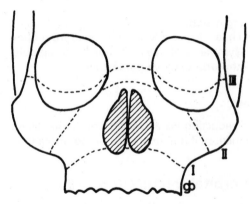

Figure 5.14 Sites for the Le Fort fracture of the middle third. The degree of symmetry varies greatly

Management

Manipulative reduction with either internal or external fixation and interdental splinting.

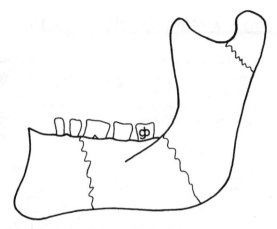

Figure 5.15 Common sites for mandibular fractures

Mandibular fractures (*Figure 5.15*)

Signs

1. Limited jaw movement due to reflex spasm.
2. Localized intra-oral tenderness.
3. Possible non-alignment of upper and lower dentition.

Management

Interdental splinting or plating.

Conclusions

- Displaced fractures can usually be diagnosed by clinical examination, especially by palpation.
- Intra-oral examination is especially important.
- Orbital involvement with diplopia and infra-orbital nerve paraesthesia are relatively common.
- Management varies depending on the stability of the reduced fragments. If unstable, wiring or packing is necessary.

Otolaryngological aspects of head injury

To many, the initial reaction must be 'What on earth have head injuries to do with ENT?' Unfortunately, this reaction reflects the present attitude regarding the role of an ENT surgeon in the management of head injuries and is to the detriment of both the patient and the medical profession. The initial aim of those managing head injuries is, naturally, to maintain the airway and ensure that the circulating blood volume is adequate. Once this has been done the general extent of injuries to the body is assessed as well as the extent and degree of damage to the head. It is to assess the latter that the ENT surgeon can be of considerable benefit as a member of a team, because it is he who can examine most competently the orifices of the skull (ear, nose, mouth) as well as assess the function of the cranial nerves, which are commonly injured as they pass through the skull foramina. This clinical examination is crucial for diagnosis as investigations, particularly radiology, do not define function. His place is just as important in the long-term management, especially in the evaluation of vertigo and hearing loss which frequently occur.

The term 'head injury' covers a range of injuries to the soft tissues of the head, the skull and its contents. Generally, but not invariably, the degree of intracranial damage is related to the extent of any skull fracture. The diagnosis and management of a patient with a head injury is thus first of the concussive effects of head injury, secondly of any fracture or its complications.

Head injury without fracture

Sudden movement of the intracranial contents within the skull cavity occasioned by a head injury, can stretch the cranial nerve fibres. Once a cranial nerve fibre has been stretched its recovery is slow and can be the cause of long-term dysfunction. Thus, the olfactory nerve is often stretched or torn at the cribriform plate and, although loss of smell at the time of injury is not often noticed because of the more dominant nature of the other complaints, it is often complained of later. The other cranial nerve that can be damaged is the audiovestibular (VIII) nerve as it leaves the brain stem to run through the internal auditory canal to innervate the cochlea and the vestibular labyrinth. A considerable proportion of individuals with a head injury, without a skull fracture, have vertigo, tinnitus or loss of hearing which can be attributed to direct damage to the VIII nerve and the end organs of hearing and balance. Alternatively, imbalance may be due to a whiplash injury to the cervical spine. The assessment of such patients is often difficult because of the emotional problems of a severe accident and frequently pending legal action. Complaints of loss of balance and hearing are most often real and should be considered seriously. Unfortunately, there is little that can be done at the time of injury to aid neural recovery and symptomatic measures are all that can be offered.

Head injury with skull fracture

Skull fractures can be either depressed or linear. Both can cause pressure symptoms by being associated with intracranial bleeding but linear fractures can, by extending some distance from the site of injury, involve the cranial nerves as they pass through the skull foramina. Fractures can involve either singly or in combination the temporal, parietal, frontal and occipital bones.

Temporal and parietal bone fractures

The temporal bone contains the ossicular chain and the end organs of hearing and balance supplied from the brain stem by the VIII cranial nerve. In addition, the temporal bone is closely integrated with the parietal bone, so that blows to the side of the head, and hence to the parietal bone, frequently involve the temporal bone. If alert enough to respond, a patient with an injury to the temporal or parietal bone may complain of dullness of hearing, disturbance of balance, tinnitus or any combination.

The diagnosis of a temporal bone fracture is clinical rather than radiological.

In assessing whether there is a temporal or parietal bone injury the area around the ear is palpated for tenderness and swelling. With time, bruising and discoloration will occur behind the ear and over the mastoid (Battle's sign). The external ear and the external auditory canal are then examined. If blood is found in the canal, and if alternative sources for this, such as lacerations, can be excluded, this is considered diagnostic of a middle cranial fossa fracture involving the temporal bone. The blood in the ear has come via a traumatic perforation of the tympanic membrane (which often cannot be seen because of the blood) from a fracture extending from the middle cranial fossa to the middle ear. A cerebrospinal fluid leak is not usually evident because of the blood, but it should be assumed to be likely.

If there is no blood in the external auditory canal, there may be blood in the middle ear (haemotympanum), evident by a blue discoloration of the tympanic membrane. This alone will give a mild conductive hearing impairment which resolves spontaneously within about four weeks. In addition, the ossicular chain may be disrupted, most often by the incus being dislocated. This results in a more severe conductive hearing impairment than a haemotympanum. If spontaneous resolution does not occur, surgical correction is required. On the other hand if the external auditory canal and the tympanic membrane are normal, a temporal bone injury cannot be excluded. In all cases pure tone audiometry must be performed as soon as the patient is cooperative. A sensorineural hearing impairment, especially of the high frequencies, is all too common.

If a fracture is suspected it is normal to prescribe prophylactic antibiotics such as penicillin and sulphadimidine to prevent intracranial infection from bacteria gaining access via the fracture line. Otherwise the management is expectant. In those with a sensorineural impairment there may be some recovery but this may take months because of the slow rate of neural regeneration. In those with disequilibrium the symptoms should also settle but again this may take many months.

On the other hand if a sensorineural impairment of vertigo is progressive, surgical exploration and packing off of the fracture line to prevent the cerebrospinal fluid leak is warranted to halt and hopefully reverse the trend.

A facial nerve palsy is a relatively uncommon complication of a temporal bone fracture but if complete and occurring immediately following the injury, warrants surgical exploration of the ear to reappose the damaged ends of the nerve.

Frontal bone fracture

The frontal sinuses are within, and the olfactory nerves pass through, the frontal bones. Stretching or tearing of the olfactory nerve can occur without a fracture, but is more frequent when there is one. With a fracture a tract is opened from the subarachnoid space to the nose, often resulting in a leak of bloody cerebrospinal fluid. This can pass unnoticed as the volume of the leak may not be large and follows the natural route of drainage from the nose via the nasopharynx to the pharynx. Sometimes, however, the patient may notice a salty taste in the mouth. It is usually only when there are copious amounts of cerebrospinal fluid that it drips via the anterior nares and becomes clinically evident. Anterior and posterior rhinoscopy should, therefore, be performed in any patient in whom a frontal bone fracture is suspected. Any watery or bloody fluid which is present is collected for analysis. The distinction of cerebrospinal fluid from a mucoid nasal discharge is most easily done by quantitative assessment of glucose, the level of this being higher in cerebrospinal fluid than in mucus. Dextrostix are often used to do this but their use is invalidated by the presence of blood, quantitative biochemical analysis then being mandatory.

Lateral radiology of the skull can on occasions delineate blood or cerebrospinal fluid levels within the frontal sinuses or intracranial air (pneumatocele) which has entered the skull via the fracture. Both of these radiological findings are considered diagnostic of a frontal bone fracture.

The management of frontal bone fracture, as of most skull fractures, is usually expectant. It is customary to prescribe prophylactic antibiotics with the aim of preventing meningitis from nasal organisms. Spontaneous closure of the cerebrospinal fluid leak is usual within ten days but if prolonged thereafter may necessitate obliteration of the frontal sinus or neurosurgical closure of the dural tear.

Occipital bone fractures

As no structures are in or pass through the occipital bone, the only complications of its fracture are intracranial. This is, therefore, the only skull bone fracture where an ENT examination does not particularly aid in diagnosis.

■ Conclusions

- A severe head injury without a skull fracture is often complicated by hearing and vestibular disorders.
- Haemotympanum or blood (and cerebrospinal fluid) in the external auditory canal is diagnostic of a middle cranial fossa fracture involving the temporal bone.
- These individuals almost invariably have a hearing loss and balance problems which may merit surgical intervention.
- A facial palsy occurring immediately following a head injury is also diagnostic of a temporal bone fracture and may merit surgical exploration.
- Loss of smell or a watery nasal discharge following a head injury suggests a frontal bone fracture.

Something stuck

Any ENT or casualty surgeon could, if he wished, build up a highly individual collection of assorted objects which have been removed from the ear, nose or throat. The majority of these will have been removed from children and, in some, it may have been a chance finding when examining the patient for a cause of otorrhoea or rhinorrhoea.

The first attempt at removal of a foreign body is always the best. Good lighting, appropriate instruments and adequate head holding especially of children, are essential. The more attempts at removal there are, the more impacted the object may become, making removal under a general anaesthetic imperative.

Something in the ear

Pencil rubbers, beads, stones, cotton wool and other objects are often poked into the external auditory canal and lost. There need not necessarily be symptoms but otorrhoea (discharging ear) is often found to be due to a piece of cotton wool lost during cleaning with a cotton bud.

All objects are best removed by non-specialists by syringing, and this includes insects, which will be drowned. There is usually a gap between the posterosuperior canal wall and the object. The water should, therefore, be aimed at the posterior canal wall in order to bypass the object and force it out with the water after being reflected from the tympanic membrane. The ear must always be examined after the object has been removed as the initial reason for poking the ear may well be underlying pathology. The other ear must also be inspected, as it often contains another object. Failed surgery requires otolaryngological removal most frequently by suction under magnification.

Something in the nose

A foreign body in the nose often remains symptomless until there is such a foul stench (*ozoena*) due to superimposed infection that parents think there must be something wrong with either the teeth or the tonsils.

Removal is achieved with the child sitting on or between the knees of a parent or nurse, with the head held upright and steady by hands

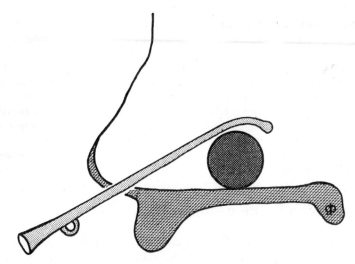

Figure 5.16 Method of removal of a nasal foreign body

placed over the ears. The foreign body usually lies on the nasal floor, lodged between the inferior turbinate and the septum. A curved blunt instrument can, therefore, be inserted over the object, which is then extracted, against the nasal floor (*Figure 5.16*).

Something in the throat

Sharp objects such as fish bones can stick anywhere in the mouth and pharynx but the areas of predilection are the tonsils, the base of the tongue, and the oropharynx. In the mouth and pharynx, as opposed to the oesophagus, patient localization of the object is reasonably accurate. Unfortunately, however, it is often difficult for the patient to differentiate between an object that remains lodged and one that has passed on. In the latter instance symptoms persist, presumably due to mild mucosa trauma. Impacted fish bones are not a danger to life, but should be removed because they are uncomfortable.

In order to identify the site of the foreign body a forehead light is essential, leaving both hands free to use the instruments. It is often better to spray the pharynx with a local anaesthetic (4 per cent lignocaine) early rather than late so that the patient's cooperation is retained. With the use of laryngeal mirrors and spatulae or tongue depressors, it should be possible to identify all objects lodged in the mouth and pharynx and remove them with angled forceps. If a foreign body cannot be identified, lateral X-rays of the neck can be helpful in localizing a radio-opaque object, fish bones sometimes coming into this category. The presence of a foreign body in the oesophagus can be suspected on mirror examination by pooling of saliva at the oesophageal inlet. Anteroposterior radiological views of the chest can be helpful in the localization of opaque objects in the oesophagus but if negative, and symptoms are present, a foreign body must be assumed.

Something in the oesophagus

Solid objects do not usually stick until they reach the oesophagus, where there are three points that are relatively narrower. The first and usual point in children is at the oesophageal inlet in the postcricoid region. The second and third sites, especially in adults, are at the arch of the aorta and the cardio-oesophageal junction where there can be associated pathology (spasm, fibrosis, stricture or neoplasm). In the elderly it is surprising what is actually swallowed and gets stuck, lumps of meat and whole segments of orange being relatively common. This is because if the elderly wear any dentures at all they often only wear the upper ones which makes it difficult for them to chew.

The management of solid objects in the oesophagus varies. Unfortunately as yet only fine forceps can be passed via a fibreoptic scope. Hence for most foreign bodies removal requires a general anaesthetic and the passing of a rigid oesophagoscope, both of which have a definite morbidity and mortality. It is not an uncommon experience to find that on passing the scope the object has spontaneously passed on in the time lapse between admission and endoscopy. The majority of oesophageal foreign bodies will do little harm so a period of observation is not dangerous but endoscopy is always performed for sharp objects because of the fear and dangers of perforation.

Endoscopy also tends to be performed earlier with large objects and in children where the hold up is at the cricopharyngeal sphincter. Otherwise, the policy is to wait and only intervene if spontaneous passage has not occurred within 24 hours. In adults it is wise to exclude any pathology, especially at the gastro-oesopha-geal junction, so if endoscopy is not carried out because the object has spontaneously passed on, a barium swallow should be subsequently performed.

■ Conclusions

- The first attempt at removal of any foreign body is always the best.
- Foreign bodies in the ear are best removed by syringing.
- Foreign bodies in the nose are best removed by a curved probe.
- Foreign bodies in the mouth and pharynx are best removed with angled forceps.
- Foreign bodies in the oesophagus can be left to see if they pass on spontaneously, unless they are sharp and likely to perforate the wall. Surgical removal is via a rigid oesophagoscope.

Appendix:
When to refer

Referral patterns to otorhinolaryngologists vary from country to country and within a country from area to area depending on the experience and facilities of the referrer and of the specialist. However, in the British context it is possible to lay down some general guidelines as to who should be referred and with what degree of urgency.

Mandatory referral within 24 hours

Uncontrollable epistaxis	To prevent death.
Stridor	To prevent death by intubation, humidification, removal of foreign body or treatment of acute epiglottitis and tumours.
Nasal and faciomaxillary trauma	For consideration of manipulation or fixation.
Facial palsy	If there is any question of otological pathology or head injury.
Sudden hearing loss	All cases in which wax or otitis media with effusion is not the cause; for assessment, monitoring and perhaps early treatment.

Mandatory referral as soon as possible

Obvious head and neck
tumours

Non-inflammatory neck lumps	To exclude a head and neck primary neoplasm.
Unilateral nasal polyps	To exclude a neoplasm.
Upper alimentary dysphagia	To exclude an oral or pharyngeal neoplasm.
Unilateral hearing impairment	To exclude a nasopharyngeal neoplasm and acoustic neuroma.

Recommended referral for investigation and management

Hearing impairment that is disabling
Disabling vertigo
Disabling tinnitus
Active chronic otitis media

Conditions not usually requiring referral

Wax
Otitis externa
Transient acute otitis media
Transient otitis media with effusion
Transient sore throats
Allergic rhinitis
Chronic sinusitis

Index